JUDY HOWARD

Bach Flower Remedies For Women

INDEX COMPILED BY LYN GREENWOOD

SAFFRON WALDEN
THE C.W. DANIEL COMPANY LIMITED

First published in Great Britain in 1992
by The C. W. Daniel Company Limited
1 Church Path, Saffron Walden
Essex, CB10 1JP, England

ISBN 0 85207 261 9

Designed by Tina Ranft
Production in association with
Book Production Consultants, Cambridge

Typeset by Rowland Phototypesetting Limited,
Bury St Edmunds, Suffolk
Printed and bound by St Edmundsbury Press Limited,
Bury St Edmunds, Suffolk

Dedicated to women everywhere but especially to

Sarah Penford

whose sincere and selfless
positivity is an example
to us all.

And Chris Ball
Lavinia Howard
Maureen Howe

Brenda Woodham
Margaret Rankin
Dawn Bainbridge

Sharon Radford
Maria Garcia
Nana and

Aunty Dot

for their experience and understanding,

and to my Mum for her warm and gentle hugs.

Contents

Introduction

In writing this book I hope to give to women the opportunity to find a way through their own personal milestones of female development by coping with, and acting positively upon, the emotional aspects of their troubles with the gentle healing benefits of the Bach Flower Remedies.

These Remedies are intended to restore our balance and equilibrium by guiding us through the negative feelings we experience and showing us the light again, so often at the end of a long dark tunnel. The Bach Remedies are safe and are helpful to everyone – adults, children, even animals and plants – selected always for the person as an individual rather than for any particular physical complaint. Dr. Bach, the Harley Street physician who discovered the Remedies during the 1930's, believed and proved to himself through extensive medical and personal research, that our emotional outlook and personality was ultimately responsible for our overall mental and physical well-being. His system of healing, therefore, is intended to treat the person rather than the disease, and therefore the cause rather than the effect.

The Bach Flower Remedies are for everyone, but can be of particular help to women because from puberty onwards, throughout a woman's reproductive life, and indeed beyond, her life is so often at the mercy of her hormones, and all the associated emotional changes that she has to cope with.

1

Rather like a roller-coaster, we step on at puberty and then finally get off when we reach the menopause, but its effects can go on long after the ride has finished.

This book is designed to consider each stage of a woman's cycle of life, and how the Bach Remedies can help ease the emotional traumas that can make those stages so trying.

About the author . . .

Judy Howard trained as a general nurse at the Queen Elizabeth Hospital in King's Lynn, Norfolk. After qualifying in 1980 she took a Staff Nurse post in the operating theatre and then gained further experience as an agency nurse in Bristol and London. In 1982 she qualified as a Midwife at the Whittington Hospital in North London and then took up a position as a secretarial and nursing assistant to a Harley Street gynaecologist obstetrician and fertility specialist of very high regard. During that time she undertook successfully a course in Family Planning and then in 1983 moved to Nottingham where she qualified as a Health Visitor and worked in the mining town of Ollerton until 1985 when she was asked if she might like to join the team at the Bach Centre. Her father, John Ramsell, had been working with Nora Weeks and Victor Bullen at Mount Vernon since 1971, and so it was a natural progression that she should join her father, and felt deeply privileged to have been offered such an opportunity.

Her role at the Bach Centre is, along with the other members of the team, to educate and offer advice about the work of Dr. Bach, and to run the teaching and training programme of the Dr. Edward Bach Foundation, the educational wing of the Bach Centre. During the summer months, she and her colleagues are busy preparing the Mother Tinctures – the Life Force and essence of the Bach Flower Remedies.

She says: "It is a great honour to be so closely involved with the work of a wonderful, yet immensely humble man; to be at Mount Vernon, his home and work-place; to sit and wander in the peaceful garden bursting with life; and to have by my side, not only my dear parents, but my husband Keith and my friend Chris whom I have known since 1977 when we met as two young and hopeful student nurses embarking on a future career together. Each day as I walk up the steps to the front door of the cottage, I most certainly count my blessings."

How The Bach System Works

The Bach Flower Remedies are intended to treat the person as an individual for the temperament and personality. They are not a treatment for physical complaints, but because our body responds either positively or negatively to the way we think and feel in ourselves, by helping us *feel* more positive our body has a chance to *respond* equally positively, and thus re-establish a general betterment in our being as a whole.

There are several books available which explain the Remedies and their uses in more detail. These are listed at the end of the book. For a comprehensive and fundamental guide to the descriptions and indications of each Remedy which is crucial to one's understanding of the system, I would recommend the following:

The Bach Flower Remedies Step by Step – this is a good all-round practical guide to the Remedies and their use, explaining how to make them part of your everyday life, using them for yourself and your family.

The Handbook of the Bach Flower Remedies – an in-depth description of each Remedy together with case histories.

Questions & Answers – a practical answer to all your questions, concerning all aspects of Dr. Bach's work.

The Twelve Healers & Other Remedies – Dr. Bach's own descriptions of the 38 Remedies.

Heal Thyself – Dr. Bach's profound yet simple philosophy of health and disease.

There are 38 Bach Flower Remedies altogether. Each one deals specifically with a particular emotional state or aspect of personality. It is a complete system because although there are many thousands of *words* to describe how we feel, when the mood or the feeling is analysed, there remain 38 fundamental states or character traits. Dr. Bach dedicated his life to researching and perfecting this approach to healing, and when he had finalised his findings he knew that his mission in life had reached its conclusion, and he then declared to his assistants Nora Weeks and Victor Bullen that his work was complete. One may wonder, if Dr. Bach were alive today, whether he would have been searching for new remedies to deal with new illnesses and the pressures of modern life, but the Remedies do not deal with these material things – they are for the emotions like fear and worry and bad temper, and for human nature itself, which remains constant throughout time and throughout the world, no matter where, how or when we might live.

The following list gives a brief indication of each Remedy for easy reference.

AGRIMONY – for those who hide their feelings behind a cheerful face.

ASPEN – for vague unknown feelings that cause apprehension and anxious anticipation.

BEECH – for those who find it hard to tolerate or understand other people's methods of doing things, and are therefore critical and easily irritated.

CENTAURY – for those who are kind and eager to please, but find their good nature easily imposed upon and exploited by those with more dominant personalities.

CERATO – for those who seek the reassurance of others as they do not trust their own decisions, judgement or intuition.

CHERRY PLUM – for irrational thoughts and fear of the mind giving way.

CHESTNUT BUD – for those who make the same mistake time and again, learning little from past experience.

CHICORY – for those inclined to impose their love on others in a selfish or possessive way, blind to their need for independence and social freedom, and who are easily hurt when snubbed.

CLEMATIS – for those who are dreamy, living in the future, day-dreaming, absent-minded, and need to have something to look forward to.

CRAB APPLE – the cleansing remedy for those who dislike themselves or feel unclean, diseased, or ugly.

ELM – for those who are normally confident but at times find the pressure and responsibility of life or work too much to cope with, and are then prone to undermine their confidence and become despondent.

GENTIAN – for depression for any known reason. For setbacks that cause discouragement or disappointment.

GORSE – for those who have lost hope of being well or of the subject of their hopelessness ever returning to normality. They are pessimistic and see only the negative outcome.

HEATHER – for those who are in need of company and companionship. They are talkative and hold on to a person's attention for as long as possible whilst they go into detail about their problems or personal life.

HOLLY – for hatred, envy, suspicion, revenge, jealousy – all the feelings that eat away at the love within us.

HONEYSUCKLE – for those whose thoughts linger in the past at the expense of their enjoyment of the present: when the mind dwells on happy memories, re-lives some unpleasant incident or yearns for how things used to be.

HORNBEAM – for those who feel they have insufficient strength to face the day ahead, or task in hand. Those who procrastinate and put things off "until tomorrow".

IMPATIENS – for those who are inclined to impatience and

irritation with slowness. They want things done in a hurry and are therefore in a hurry themselves.

LARCH – for those who lack confidence in their ability: those who do not believe in themselves, are afraid of failure and so do not try.

MIMULUS – for those who are afraid and lack courage. For everyday, known fears, and for those who are shy, or timid.

MUSTARD – for depression for no apparent reason. An unhappiness that descends and then lifts like a passing cloud but without an identifiable cause.

OAK – for those who have an inner strength – the plodders who soldier on through life despite its pitfalls.

OLIVE – for tiredness, fatigue, exhaustion. When one has been working hard, studying or concentrating and feels drained as a result.

PINE – for those who feel guilty and blame themselves, even for something that was not their fault: harbouring a guilt complex or have a guilty conscience from which they are unable to set themselves free.

RED CHESTNUT – for those who are afraid for the safety and well-being of those they care about: over-anxious and fearful.

ROCK ROSE – for terror, panic, nightmares and other fears of a horrifying nature.

ROCK WATER – for those who are strict with themselves, set themselves high standards and targets and demand perfection of their efforts.

SCLERANTHUS – for those who are indecisive, debating the pro's and con's of every situation – hesitating "shall I, shan't I?"

STAR OF BETHLEHEM – for shock, the effects of serious news, bereavement, sorrow and grief.

SWEET CHESTNUT – for utter despair – heartbreaking anguish as though there is no end in sight.

VERVAIN – for those who are incensed by injustice. They speak out to make their point known, try to persuade others to believe in what they have to say. They work hard, enthusiastic in all they embark upon, and are prone to become tense and highly stressed.

VINE – for those who are of a strong and dominant nature. The leaders who are tempted to use their position and strength to control others, taking no notice of their feelings or preferences, demanding obedience and acceptance of their orders.

WALNUT – the remedy for change and any period of adjustment when one feels unsettled, and for those who are influenced or distracted by the influence of others.

WATER VIOLET – for those who are reserved, self-contained, dignified people who enjoy peace and quiet. May become "cut off" due to their need for privacy and may therefore appear aloof or unapproachable.

WHITE CHESTNUT – for worrying thoughts and mental arguments that interfere with rest and peace of mind.

WILD OAT – for those who are at a cross-roads in life and do not know in which direction they should proceed. They tend to feel unfulfilled and dissatisfied with what they have achieved, and have ambitions to do something of value.

WILD ROSE – for those who are unmotivated and resigned to all that happens. Not interested in change: happy with life the way it is. For apathy and resignation or feelings of staleness.

WILLOW – for resentment or bitterness. For those who find it hard to forgive and forget, but dwell on negativity and their own misfortunes.

RESCUE REMEDY – a combination of Star of Bethlehem, Rock Rose, Clematis, Cherry Plum and Impatiens. The composite for emergencies – accidents, examination nerves etc. Its all-round calming properties are comforting in a crisis. Rescue Remedy can also be applied to the skin to remove the shock and subsequent pain from an area following a knock or minor burn. Rescue Remedy Cream (which also contains Crab Apple for its cleansing properties) is also very soothing for external application and as it is a general healing salve, can be applied to abrasions, bruises, skin irritations etc.

The descriptions of the Remedies above have been given for their indications which is why the moods have been put in negative terms. There is, however, a positive aspect to them all – effectively, the opposite of the negative – and this is what you are striving to achieve by taking the remedy that is indicated. For a good, down to earth, description of both negative and positive aspects, and thus a balanced approach to each Remedy, I would suggest *The Dictionary of the Bach Flower Remedies*, by Tom Hyne-Jones.

You will note that as well as the Remedies being descriptive of moods and states of mind common to most of us from time to time, there are those that are descriptive of character traits, types of people and personalities. When choosing remedies it is important not only to select remedies that relate to the mood, but also to the personality. In other words, put the moods into context with your natural disposition, thereby treating yourself as a **whole person**.

A few remedies can be given at a time, depending on your needs, up to about six or seven. They are quite harmless and so no overdose or conflict can occur. They can be taken quite safely with other medication, and because they are benign in their action will not interfere with other treatments you may be taking. The Remedies are however, preserved in brandy and so it is recommended that they are diluted in water as follows: having chosen your remedies, put 2 drops of each one into a bottle of approximately 30ml (1oz) size (a smaller bottle will do just as well if necessary). Then fill up with water (mineral water is the most suitable because it will remain fresh for longer than tap water). Then, from this prepared bottle, take 4 drops at least 4 times daily, or more often if required.

As an alternative, the drops can be added to a glass of water and sipped at intervals during the day, and this may be more convenient if the remedies are simply to help you overcome a passing mood. As an on-going treatment and for deep-seated problems however, it is more economical and usually more convenient to make a composite treatment bottle.

Rescue Remedy is extremely helpful in emergency situations and it can be taken as and when required – 4 drops in a little water, or neat from the bottle if no liquid is to hand.

This book provides a comprehensive guide to how the Bach Flower Remedies can be of help to women. As we explore each potentially problematic phase, we will be discussing the Remedies in more detail and relating them to all aspects of womanhood. Dr. Bach wanted us all to accept the Remedies as a natural part of our lives. I hope that with the help of this book, the Remedies will become a natural part of **your** life, helping to enrich it so that you are able to experience or re-capture the true beauty and joy of being a woman.

CHAPTER ONE

Woman's View Of Herself

Let us begin by considering our body – our looks and figure. Women come in all shapes and sizes – short, tall; petite, heavy; flat chested, buxom, to name but a few. As young children, shape and size seems to matter very little. Friendship, and therefore personality is, by and large, the important issue. Children who are good at games, funny, extrovert and friendly tend to be the popular ones at school. Appearances seem to become more important as the child gets older, and there is then a need for the individual to belong and fit in. Collectively, children often tend to single out a "misfit" in the class or school, a child who seems different and therefore stands out from the rest. Being too fat or too thin; too unkempt or too smart; too bright or too slow – anything that makes a child the odd one out. For whatever reason children are snubbed, they are faced with having to either accept it and put up with the teasing and friendlessness, or try to win the favour of their peers by proving that they are worth knowing. This might rest with achievement at sport, or by making everyone else laugh, by organizing a prank or being the life and soul of the classroom. The other children will then be more interested in the personality of the child and forget about what may otherwise have been the subject of ridicule.

As we move into our teens, appearances tend to become more important. Adults generally appreciate that there is more to a person than what is first seen, but it is not until we really get to know a person that a true opinion can be formed. Sometimes there is a temptation to make up our minds at first glimpse, and this frequently happens when being introduced to a prospective new boyfriend, meeting someone new at a party or night club, or going on a blind date. Most people I am sure will be able to recall some incident or occasion when they have taken an instant dislike to someone, having based their opinion on appearances alone. I can remember as a teenager being very fussy about the looks of the boys I went out with, and I am sure there are many women who, like me, have danced with a seemingly handsome man in a dimly lit discotheque and then, although perhaps ashamed to admit it, feeling utterly disappointed when the lights were switched on at the end of the evening! Thankfully, as we grow up and become adults, we begin to take more notice of what lies beneath the surface and less of what is superficial. Nevertheless, often we have a pre-conceived idea of what our ideal partner should look like, and this can get in the way of our appreciation of a person's finer qualities or prevent us really getting to know them properly. Beauty is, after all, only skin deep, and if we would just take the trouble to look inside and explore, we might find a host of hidden treasures that are much more beautiful and that will radiate through the outer casing given the chance.

When we consider how we perceive other people, it is easier to understand how we perceive ourselves. The reason for self-dissatisfaction, vanity, self-approval or disapproval becomes clearer. Often the same criteria we use to measure the standards of others apply to self-examination, and so we may find that we criticize others for what we do not like in ourselves. This applies to physical appearance as well as to faults in the character. It is however, regard for oneself that matters when it comes to enjoying life uninhibited. If we have a positive regard for ourselves then we feel comfortable with our being and can get on with living, unhindered by self-absorbing thoughts about what other people might think of us. This is often easier said than done however, and for most women there is usually something they dislike about themselves or have a hang-up about, whether it is noticeable

11

or not, and inevitably there will be someone else who would consider it a blessing to be endowed with such "faults". If we could swap features like we might swap stamps, perhaps we would all be happy! Or perhaps not . . .

Come what may, we do what we can to enhane what we **do** have – wearing flattering clothes, make-up, or adopting a new hair-style are all ways and means of making us feel better, and are as much for our own benefit as for that of others. Looking good makes us feel good, and when we feel good we feel happy. It is, therefore, therapeutic to take an interest in ourselves, and so a little self-indulgent pampering once in a while by treating oneself to a day at a health and beauty club is a tremendously revitalising experience and can truly work wonders!

To be acceptable to ourselves, therefore, is a good reason for attending to physical appearance, but would we always take so much trouble if we lived in isolation far away from anyone, like a recluse? Would it matter then what we looked like? Who would see? Most women in this situation would probably stop wearing make-up, choose to wear comfortable clothes without thinking about coordinated outfits or worrying about how well the colours matched, or, for that matter, whether they had even been ironed! Some women, on the other hand, would make sure they looked immaculate no matter what, either to satisfy their own needs, or "just in case" they had an unexpected visitor. On the whole, it would seem that our personal appearance matters the most when there is someone else to appreciate it. It may be those who feature strongly in our lives – boyfriend, husband, lover for example, or because we want to indicate a position of authority or look efficient. Of course, we do not always try to look good for men, women dress up for other women too – fashion itself provokes competition. By and large, we tend to want to project an image or recognition for other people to see, no matter who they are, but at the end of the day, we judge ourselves; how we look either meets with our own approval or it does not.

OUR BODY, OUR FIGURE AND DIETING

Very few women are completely satisfied with their figure. Someone who is thin may envy those who are more rounded, and likewise, those with fuller figures may give anything to be thin. Or there may be just one part of our body that we dislike – perhaps our thighs seem a little too chunky or our bust too small or too large. Some women pursue a surgical approach to reduce their fatty areas or to change the shape of their nose or size of their breasts. Cosmetic surgery however, is not always related to vanity. There are occasions when it is done to improve the quality of a person's life, due to a disfigurement for example that causes a great amount of distress, and this could apply to anything from a bad scar to protruding ears.

Cosmetic surgery however, is an extreme measure in most instances. Where weight is concerned, prevention is undoubtedly better than cure, and although it is a lot easier said than done, if it can be controlled, then the unpleasant side effects associated with obesity will not occur. Food is the body's fuel. We need it to enable our organs to function properly, to give us energy so that we can live healthily. What our body needs however, and what it gets, are two different things and do not by any means always coincide! The body needs a well-balance diet – one that contains a proportion of protein, carbohydrates, fats and fibre, together with an adequate intake of all the essential vitamins and minerals. It is the right proportion of each one that is, for a lot of people, difficult to achieve.

Energy is measured in calories, the unit value given to food. Those which provide calories in high proportions and thus foods which will readily be converted and used for energy are carbohydrates; starches, sugars and fats. If the calorific intake is greater than the body's energy requirements, the excess will be stored as fat. Some women use energy at a faster rate than others and thus require more calories than those who have a slower metabolism. Similarly, women who take a lot of physical exercise or who are working in a job that involves a lot of walking – nurses, policewomen, traffic wardens etc – will also require a diet

13

that will provide more energy than those in more sedentary occupations. However, the brain uses a vast amount of energy, and so a person who works at a desk involved in mentally taxing work, may be using up more energy than someone who has a more physically demanding occupation.

If the diet is well-balanced, consuming fattening foods in moderation in proportions suited to our own needs, and taking plenty of fresh raw foods, fruit and vegetables, there should be no need for any of us to embark on a specific weight loss programme. If a person is overweight then, apart from certain endocrine disorders which would require specialised treatment, it is usually due to either over-eating or lack of exercise, and both cases are correctable with a little, or perhaps a lot, of motivation. In most instances, attention in both areas is required. For those who do need to lose weight, dieting should be taken gradually. It is no use going on a crash diet that will shed the excess weight too quickly, because although in the short term it makes one feel pleased and gives encouragement, it invariably causes the body to "clamp down". If a dramatically reduced diet is forthcoming, then the body, having been used to a greater quantity of food, suddenly finds itself having to draw on its store of fat for conversion to energy, no longer being able to rely on the food intake to cater for its needs. This brings about the initial speedy reduction in weight, but once the body has got over the shock of being caught unawares, it puts on the brakes. Metabolism slows down and the body begins to hold onto its reserves, finding a way to utilise only the food that is provided for essentials and so preserving its store.

It is this compensatory action that slows down the weight loss, and although an even further reduction in food consumption will inevitably win the battle, it can only be temporary because as soon as normal eating habits are resumed, the body's own survival instincts come into play, and as a defence, it begins to build up an even bigger store of reserve energy than ever before! As a result, the weight gain, unless it is closely monitored, will become even greater, resulting in the disheartening realisation that there has been a big step forward but two even bigger steps back. It is therefore essential when embarking on a weight loss programme to not only take regular exercise to force the body to draw on its energy resources, but to diet gently and gradually. It will take longer but will be far more effective in the long term. If you feel impatient with this slow process, **IMPATIENS** is the remedy to help. If you feel discouraged, have suffered a set-back or feel disheartened and unsuccessful, then **GENTIAN** will give you the encouragement to persevere with restored optimism. **GORSE** will restore hope if you feel totally pessimistic. For those who know they should lose weight, but keep putting it off and tell themselves, as they tuck into another slice of cake, "I'll start my diet tomorrow", **HORNBEAM** is the remedy to ensure that "tomorrow" does actually come! If you have had several attempts, but have reverted back to old eating habits and consequently put on excess weight again, then **CHEST-NUT BUD** would be helpful as this will help you to learn from your experience and use it to remind you if you should drift into temptation too frequently!

Dieting can, however, become an obsession, and this applies to those who really need to lose weight as well as those who need to lose very little if any at all. It is the poor self-image which stimulates the desire to improve one's looks by dieting, but it can be taken to extremes and may cause, in some women, an obsessional neurosis whereby they do not see themselves as they really are, but as an ugly, out of shape and grotesque configuration of their true being. **CRAB APPLE** is the remedy to deal with such feelings as it helps to improve that self image, helps you to respect and like yourself so that you can look in the mirror and feel comfortable with what you see, instead of disgust at some distorted reflection. **ROCK WATER** is also a helpful remedy to consider for the rigidity of the strict regime and unbending self-denial. There may also be a great lack of self-confidence for which **LARCH** would be indicated.

Anorexia is commonly interpreted as the "slimmers' disease". This is a slightly misleading notion because although it can be caused by over-zealous dieting which gets out of control, it is not by any means always the case. Many women suffering with this condition do not have a weight problem but simply do not like themselves, or have a desire to punish themselves for some reason. Again **CRAB APPLE** is the remedy to help here. There are others who find food repellant or dirty and cannot bear to eat it. This again would indicate **CRAB APPLE** for the sense of contamination. **HOLLY** may also help as often there is suspicion of what damage the food might do, or of the motives of the person who has prepared it. There may be guilt at being "such a nuisance" in which case **PINE** would be called for. In fact, there could be numerous reasons, most of which are deep rooted, and so careful and delicate counselling is needed to help the sufferer open up sufficiently to enable the correct selection of Remedies to be made.

The above condition is Anorexia Nervosa, but there is a sister condition called Anorexia Bulimia, where food may be taken in secret binges and then afterwards, when a feeling of self-disgust becomes overwhelming, the food is vomited. Once again, it is the causes that are important as far as the Bach Flower Remedies are concerned, but as with Anorexia Nervosa, there tends to be a great deal of self-hatred, self-disgust and self-punishment for which **CRAB APPLE** is important. However, although in a number of cases the causal focus is on oneself, it may be quite the reverse. It may be due to deep-seated resentment or hatred of other members of the family – parents, guardians, for example, and the self-destructive behaviour is performed as a means of expressing that anger. **HOLLY** is the remedy for this hatred, or **WILLOW** for resentment. **HOLLY** would also help ease feelings of jealousy, due to sibling rivalry for example.

There is another group of people who may suffer with either complaint, who have suffered some sort of emotional trauma in a fundamental relationship with their parents and who have, as a result, so little self-confidence or self-worth that they subconsciously draw attention to themselves through self-inflicted injury, by focusing on their eating habits in an attempt to gain attention and compensate for the devotion and love that is missing. **STAR OF BETH-LEHEM** is the remedy to help ease that sense of loss; **CHICORY** for holding on, possessiveness, and needing attention; **CERATO** for those who seek reassurance from others; **WILLOW** for those who dwell on their misfortune and unhappy circumstances; **HEATHER** for self-absorption. For those who hide the way they feel, or try to hide their wasted body, **AGRIMONY** is a valuable remedy to ease the inner pain and torture. For those who are afraid of food, **MIMULUS** would help, or **ROCK ROSE** if there is actual terror. Eating a meal in front of other people can also be extremely traumatic. **LARCH** would give more confidence to those who feel self-conscious about eating in public. **PINE** is the remedy to help those who feel guilty about not being able to finish their meal, and **MIMULUS** for those who develop a fear of eating at all. This aspect alone may get out of proportion and a dread of choking, for example, may follow. **ROCK ROSE** would help ease such a terrifying ordeal. Because so many different remedies may be indicated, it is therefore extremely important that the personality of the individual is taken into account. As with any other problem, as far as the Bach Remedies are concerned, one cannot generalize, and so although there may be common features in a number of people suffering with either anorectic condition, there are always reasons and emotions individual to each one, and so each case must be assessed accordingly.

Our figure and our looks are central to the way we view ourselves. They are what give us confidence and self-assurance. However, it is not only our size or shape that matters. Whilst getting ready for work or to go out, the sense of "not feeling right" is a familiar one to most women. When the clothes we put on look drab or inappropriate, it makes us feel uncomfortable. Some mornings, looking in the mirror, one's face might look fresh and wide-eyed and would pass happily without make-up, yet other mornings, one looks in the same mirror and sees a blotchy skin, saggy cheeks and puffy eyes and would not even consider walking out of the door bare-faced! At times like these, other women who always seem to look good whatever they wear – hair shiny, posture well balanced, eyelashes long and dark – seem infinitely more attractive.

It is, however, all relative. For what is one woman's downfall is another woman's virtue, and there are unseen qualities to make up for any physical imperfections. A sense of humour, gentleness, kindliness and a warm smile are aspects of beauty that go far deeper than an unblemished skin or trim figure, and far longer lasting than those applied with a make-up brush or tube of hair colour. These aspects of a woman's being are what brings her to life, and ultimately what others are attracted to – the substance of the cake itself, not just its icing.

SEXUALITY

In adolescence

Coming to terms with one's sexuality begins in childhood with curiosity about what makes males different from females; what makes women different from girls and men from boys. What follows is a natural progression to questioning the facts of life. At one time, anything to do with sex was a taboo subject, and consequently women grew up in ignorance of the significance of their bodily changes. Girls were frightened when their period started, believing that they must be bleeding to death because nobody had warned them of what to expect, and they were not informed enough to recognize its meaning. Sometimes women got married knowing nothing of the male anatomy or of how babies are made. In some instances the man was none the wiser either, and I am aware of marriages which have tragically never been consumated simply because the couple did not know what to do.

Thankfully each generation has become more broad minded and appreciative of the need for young people to receive answers to these fundamental questions about life. These days, sex education is part of the school curriculum and begins at an early stage, in some areas during primary education. Yet, despite being equipped with the knowledge of the sexual development that takes place between childhood and mature adulthood, girls in particular are frequently embarrassed when puberty commences – when their chest starts to develop and they begin to grow hair in personal areas of their anatomy. Some adolescent girls will go to great lengths to try and hide their body, perhaps by wearing a tight vest so that their developing breasts do not show. For others it may be a time of joy, and they are proud of their new womanly figure and look forward to growing up. However, once again, it is being "normal" that really matters – the need for acceptance by peers and not feeling the odd one out. A well developed girl may be pleased with her physical pre-cociousness if she has a friend who is similarly developed, but otherwise might be acutely embarrassed and ashamed of herself, perhaps even the object of ridicule if she happened to be the only one in her age group wearing a bra or having periods. Similarly, an underdeveloped girl may feel "abnormal" if she is the only one still physically immature. Here again, even at this age, self-image is influenced by the opinion and standards of other people.

The next stage of development during adolescence after the initial physical changes have taken place at puberty, is that of emotional growth. Self consciousness and embarrassment about one's body and about what other people think of it, is often the first hurdle to overcome. **LARCH** is a helpful remedy as it allows confidence to grow. For those who are over-concerned with their appearance, and for those who think about it constantly, other remedies are indicated. **CRAB APPLE** for those who are obsessed with some detail about themselves that they do not like; **HEATHER** for those wrapped up in self-glorification, unable to consider others, talking only about themselves; or **CHICORY** for the desire to be the centre of attention.

During this particular growth period, self-awareness leads to self exploration – a period of learning about oneself. This is a normal and wholly natural pattern and not one to feel guilty or ashamed about. However, for girls who are, **CRAB APPLE** is for the sense of shame of self disgust, and **PINE** if there is a feeling of guilt, believing she has done something wrong. Adolescence is a period of discovery – getting to know ourselves, coming to terms with who we are and acknowledging our sexual identity. This in itself can present problems during these transitional years. Girls and boys of pre-pubescent age are, usually, closer to friends of the same sex. This friendship pattern continues throughout life, but as one gets older and develops feelings of sexual attraction, one becomes drawn, more intimately, to members of the opposite sex. However, before this happens, during the learning process of youth, the sexual urges which occur during puberty may be expressed and explored with friends of the same sex, those we are naturally close to. These feelings, at the time, are not clearly understood, but the curiosity and need for experimentation are there all the same. Many young people who have been involved in pre-adolescent activities with members of the same sex may become worried that they might be homosexual. These activities are more common than one might think however, and a normal part of growing up. Indeed, most young people who have experimented this way and have embarked on some sort of pre-adolescent exploration with a friend of the same gender, grow up to lead normal happy heterosexual lives.

It is therefore, during adolescence when the emotional aspect of our sexuality begins. We start seeing boys and then men in a different light, and again, there is the curiosity factor – what is it like to kiss etc. – tinged, to a certain extent, with apprehension and nervousness – what will I say to him? will he like me? what if I embarrass myself by my naivety? Television programmes, magazines and the media generally tend to whet our appetite for what is to come, and with the added peer-group pressure, it is not surprising that many young people find themselves experiencing sex before they might intuitively feel ready. Depending on the circumstances under which it took place, there may be repercussions and regrets later on.

Let us examine a few of the most commonly troublesome issues first:

FEAR　This can be divided into known and unknown fears and then sub-divided into lesser and greater extremes. For known fears of a general day-to-day nature, **MIMULUS** is the remedy indicated – fear of pregnancy, fear of contracting a sexually transmitted disease, fear of blood, pain or being injured. Vaguer fears of a less obvious nature – a sense of fear, anxiousness, apprehension and so on are dealt with by the remedy **ASPEN**. For terror and horrifying fears **ROCK ROSE** would apply, and for uncontrollable fears, a too vivid imagination that allows the fear to take charge and run riot, **CHERRY PLUM** is the indicated remedy.

SENSITIVITY   **LARCH** for feelings of inadequacy or for fear of failure or being a let-down; **WALNUT** for protection against people's interference – for those who are easily influenced by the ideas and forceful pressure or opinions of others, often against their better judgement; **CERATO** for those who need to be reassured, feeling uncertain about their judgement and reasoning – those who ask advice from others and find it hard to listen to their own intuition; **CENTAURY** for those who are easily dominated or imposed upon – those who are weak-willed and find it easier to go along with what others desire than to stand up for themselves and say "no"; **AGRIMONY** for those who pretend to be enjoying themselves, gaily going along with the crowd, when really they are hating every minute; **STAR OF BETHLEHEM** for shock.

SELF-REPROACH   **PINE** for feelings of guilt for having done something wrong, or believing that to be the case even if it is not so; **CRAB APPLE** for self-disgust or a feeling of having had one's body violated; **CENTAURY** for disappointment with oneself for being weak and succumbing to dominance.

WORRY   **WHITE CHESTNUT** for mental arguments, persistent thoughts going round in the mind, causing restlessness and insomnia in some instances. Worry might be interlinked with

21

another emotion – based on fear or guilt for example, in which case the appropriate remedy such as Mimulus or Pine would be taken in addition. For those who suffer inwardly and find it hard to confide in parents, siblings etc., **AGRIMONY** would be helpful for the turbulent emotions, but the personality as a whole should always be considered in order to put the mood and reasons for it into context. For parents who worry and are afraid for the welfare of their children **RED CHESTNUT** will help to soothe that anxious mind.

In adulthood

Having discussed some of the traumas associated with growing up, let us now turn our attention to those associated with adulthood. Relationships are a central feature in most people's lives and the traumatic ups and downs of love can go from one extreme to the other. A whole range of emotions are to be expected at some time during one relationship or another, from ecstasy to utter misery. Other, but no less intense emotions can be the result of shattered dreams of a prospective association or of desperate longing to meet someone with whom a loving relationship will develop. Whatever emotions are raised and for whatever reasons, it may be safely said that men, love, sex and marriage play a major part in a woman's life and therefore have an important influence on her sexuality and identity.

We will be discussing some problems associated with sex in Chapter Six but it would seem appropriate here, to address some inbred attitudes that can have a profound impact on adult life. Sociological factors, and in particular parental influence can affect a woman's understanding and balanced awareness of the fundamental facts of life and of her own personal sexuality. Despite the drift towards a more open-minded approach and freedom of information in today's society, old habits tend to die hard. Prudishness of parents, for example, may be transferred to their children, who may in turn grow up with a similar outlook; Victorian attitudes about morality may be passed on from one generation to the next. To help relax such rigid ideas, **ROCK WATER** would be a useful remedy, as such ideas so often belong to those who are hard task masters on themselves and therefore demand similar standards from other members of the family. **VINE** would also be helpful for the dominance, demanding conformity. If children have a very strict upbringing in this way, the values and moral judgements they place on life as they grow up are frequently coloured by those of their parents, and fear may prevent any deviation taking place. Religious beliefs may also impose strict adherence to a certain way of life, and here again fear and lack of autonomy may be part of the problem. This is not to say that such religious principles are wrong, but simply that they have the potential, in some instances, to rule rather than guide. Here again **ROCK WATER** is helpful to soften the harshness of such a strict approach. If fear is a problem then **MIMULUS** would be helpful, and **CENTAURY** if the gentleness of the personality is too easily dominated, to such an extent that this type of person finds it hard to live her own life. For those who are uncertain or hesitant about what to do or what to believe, **SCLERANTHUS** is the remedy to ease this dilemma. Sometimes guilt stands in the way of progress – feeling guilty for considering other opportunities, or for going against the expectations of parents or the Church. **PINE** is the remedy to ease the burden of self-incrimination. **WALNUT** is a helpful remedy during any transitional period, and as it acts as a link breaker, is helpful in maintaining protection from the influence of others that may interfere with progress along one's own intended path in life.

> "Parents should be particularly on guard against any desire to mould the young personality according to their own ideas or wishes, and should refrain from any undue control or demand of favours in return for their natural duty and divine privilege of being the means of helping a soul to contact the world. Any desire for control, or wish to shape the young life for personal motives; if there is the least desire to dominate, it should be checked at the onset. . . . Such should be the attitude of parent to child, giving care, love and protection as far as may be

needed and beneficial, yet never for one moment interfering with the natural evolution of the personality, as
this must be dictated by the Soul."

Edward Bach, Heal Thyself, 1931

CHAPTER TWO

Menstruation And The Reproductive Cycle

In this chapter we will be examining the normal workings of the female body, and in particular the reproductive system since it is that, and its related functions, which are responsible for most of our difficulties!

In order to understand **why** these differences occur, we need first of all to understand some straightforward anatomy. The human body is extremely complex, but it divides neatly into various systems – the respiratory system, circulatory system, digestive system, skeletal system and so on – and so if we isolate the area upon which we wish to concentrate, it becomes much simpler and easier to understand.

The female reproductive system's main focal point is on the organs within the pelvis – the uterus (or womb) and the ovaries – but for these organs to function normally, input from other areas of the body is required, and in particular from the pituitary gland situated at the base of the brain which provides the ovaries with the correct signals for it to propagate and release mature ova. The ovaries in turn, send out their own signals to encourage other parts of the reproductive system to respond – the lining of the uterus, the cervix and the breasts. All the changes that take place during

THE FEMALE REPRODUCTIVE ORGANS

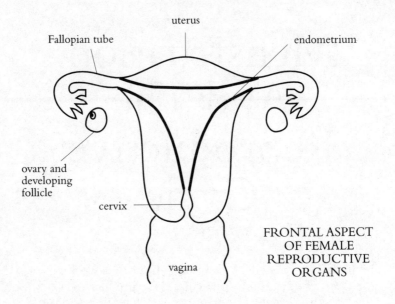

uterus

Fallopian tube

endometrium

ovary and
developing
follicle

cervix

vagina

FRONTAL ASPECT
OF FEMALE
REPRODUCTIVE
ORGANS

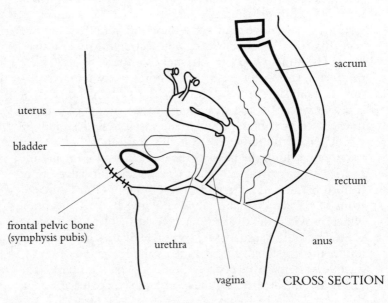

sacrum

uterus

bladder

rectum

frontal pelvic bone
(symphysis pubis)

urethra

anus

vagina

CROSS SECTION

the cycle are in preparation for a pregnancy. If it does not occur, then the whole cycle starts all over again.

These events are more easily explained in terms of a diagram as shown on the following page.

The smooth functioning of the entire reproductive system is totally reliant on the correct messages being transmitted, received and acted upon. If we imagine it in terms of radio transmission, the sound network is dependent on the transmitter and the correct signals being transmitted. Any breakdown that causes interference of these signals affects the whole system – just as a radio in your kitchen is quite useless if there is a transmission failure or the sound waves are so weak that reception is inaudible. The "radio transmitter" of our reproductive system is the area of the brain called the hypothalamus. The "signal director" is the pituitary gland which acts on the signals received from the hypothalamus. The "sound waves" are the hormones which carry messages to the "receiver" – the ovary.

There are several hormones that have a part to play, but the starring roles are provided by four main hormones – Follicle Stimulating Hormone (FSH) which is released from the pituitary gland to the ovary which causes the primary follicle to develop and prepare for ovulation, Oestrogen which is produced by the follicle and causes the lining of the uterus (endometrium) to thicken, Luteinising Hormone which is released by the pituitary gland in response to the increase in oestrogen, stimulating ovulation within about 24–36 hours of its release. This hormone also acts upon the follicle, now void of its ovum, to fill it with a yellow substance called corpus luteum. Corpus luteum produces progesterone which increases the blood supply to the endometrium so that it becomes engorged with blood and capable of sustaining the implantation of a fertilized ovum. The corpus luteum produces progesterone for fourteen days. If no pregnancy has occured by this time, it degenerates, the levels of progesterone and oestrogen fall and the lining of the uterus is shed.

This cycle of events repeats itself each month, taking approximately 28 days to complete. The cycle begins at puberty around the age of twelve and goes on, month after

THE MENSTRUAL CYCLE & DEVELOPMENT OF THE OVARIAN FOLLICLE

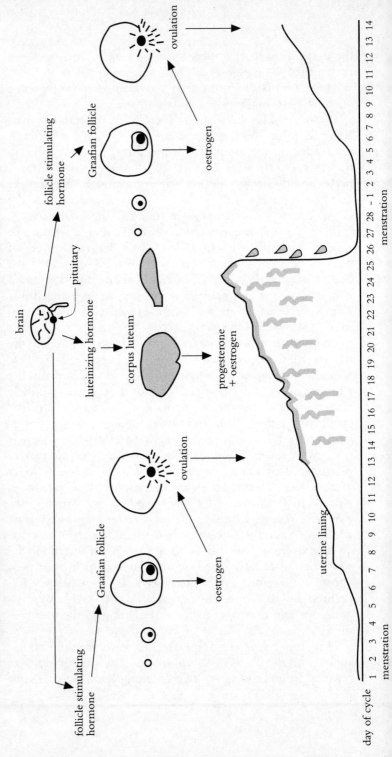

month, until the menopause or climacteric at around the age of 50.

These are a woman's childbearing years, and during each cycle there is potential for a new life to begin. A woman's ovary contains many thousands of egg cells which are there from birth, but during each cycle, some begin to ripen until one is mature enough to be released from the ovary to try its luck at becoming a new human being! On most occasions it is a vain attempt because out of some 4–500 monthly cycles over the 40 or so fertile years, it succeeds on an average of 2–3 occasions, thanks to modern methods of contraception! Of course many other factors have to coincide, and these will be discussed in more detail when we consider fertility and infertility in the next chapter.

In the meantime, let us turn our attention to the normal menstrual cycle with all its disturbances and how it can have a severe effect on some women **all** the time, others only some of the time, and a few (although I have yet to discover one!), never suffering with symptoms at all!

PRE-MENSTRUAL TENSION

During the period after ovulation and before the menstrual period begins, the hormones are reaching their peak, and this hormonal activity can cause a disturbance within our entire system. Women generally become more sensitive or "emotional" at this time and many suffer with negative emotional symptoms – hence the term "pre-menstrual tension", and these feelings are often accompanied by physical symptoms too. This combination is called "pre-menstrual syndrome".

We are all individuals and so each woman will experience slightly different disturbances during this phase of the cycle. Our usual personality and temperament play an important part too, because during the pre-menstrual phase, we are at our most vulnerable and so the surge of negative moods represents an imbalance in the even keel of our natural disposition. A tilt occurs to upset the emotional see-saw, and before we know it, a snowballing effect has started.

Most commonly, pre-menstrual symptoms include depression, irritability, intolerance and lethargy. Everything seems to get on the nerves and so one becomes short tempered and impatient with those around. So often it is those whom we care most about – our husband, partner, children, parents or close friends – that get the brunt of our bad feelings and so they too may need some help with the Remedies! Frequently there is a loss of all rationality and an inability to explain **why** we should feel the way we do – the whole package of emotional symptoms just seems to descend and take control of our feelings, leaving us helpless to resist. It is a matter of taking stock and waiting for it to pass. The problem, however is that two weeks is an awfully long time to feel like a volcano about to erupt, and an even longer time for the person who happens to be the one about to be scorched by the hot flow of lava!

On so many occasions, the smallest irritation can ignite the flame. One may feel oneself becoming irritated, but cannot control the emotion, and so inevitably there is an explosion. It is, without doubt, a difficult period for everyone concerned. The whole trying time can be eased tremendously if you have an understanding partner, but if neither of you know **why** you are behaving the way you do, then it can be extremely difficult to come to terms with. All too often an angry scene erupts which can have disastrous repercussions for any relationship if it goes on and on, leaving a trail of animosity in its wake which may, in itself, create a wedge between you. At the other extreme, a most understanding partner may provoke even more irritation because there is no response to your outburst – no ignition – and so the volcano begins to simmer with frustration . . . Then, when it is all over, when the menstrual flow brings relief from all the tension, so feelings of guilt may begin to set in when the woman reflects on how she has behaved, what she has said and the hearts she has broken – not to mention the vases, dinner plates, cups, saucers . . . !

This sudden onslaught of feelings can be quite overwhelming, if not alarming, but the Bach Remedies really can help. They are gentle and subtle but very effective, and they are there to help us cope with these emotions and help us to rise above them, not have our lives dictated to or controlled by the power of a bad mood. As explained earlier, the Bach

Remedies are chosen on a very individual basis. It is impossible to generalise and provide a "pre-menstrual mix" suitable
for all women. We are all different and so our own personal
combination will vary. There are nevertheless, some symptoms that are common to most, and so the Remedies that are
listed here would generally be helpful to consider.

For the period of adjustment . . .
WALNUT
This remedy is for adjustment to change. It is helpful during
any transitional period which may include moving house,
settling into a new job or new area, or through the major
milestone changes of life such as teething, puberty, pregnancy and menopause. It is therefore often a helpful remedy
during the menstrual cycle because this again is a period of
adjustment due to body changes in preparation for reproduction. Walnut, being the link-breaker helps to stabilize and
bridge the gap during these changes evening out the humps
and dips of the menstrual cycle's roller-coaster track.

For depression . . .
MUSTARD
This remedy is for the type of depression that descends like a
dark cloud for no apparent reason. It casts a shadow of gloom
on the sufferer and while it is there, life is without joy. It is
like a lead weight inside – each day becomes a drudgery; one
goes through the motions, but with a heavy heart. This is
typically the sort of depression that accompanies pre-
menstrual tension in some women, and in such instances, the
remedy can bring a wonderful relief to this awful unhappiness, driving the cloud away and allowing the sunshine to
reappear.

For irritability . . .
IMPATIENS
This remedy, as its name suggests, is for impatience, irritability and short-temper. There is an "Impatiens type" of
person who is naturally impatient with slowness, preferring
to work at her own pace to prevent being hindered by the
slowness of others. If you are of this nature normally then

during the pre-menstrual phase of your cycle, this tendency is likely to be more exaggerated, but it is a common feeling in most women at this time and the remedy can therefore help us all should we feel this way.

For intolerance . . .
BEECH
This remedy is similar to Impatiens in a way, but is more for an intolerance of people; criticizing their failings, short-comings and so on. The "Beech type" is one who finds it hard to understand what, to them, appears to be stupidity in other people. They find it hard to place themselves in the shoes of another and do not suffer "fools" gladly. This frame of mind, like that of the "Impatiens type" is extremely common during the pre-menstrual phase, when everyone and everything gets on one's nerves, one is finding fault with those around, and the little things that would hardly be noticed normally become increasingly annoying. Beech helps us to be more relaxed and understanding with our family and friends – and everyone else for that matter!

For irrational thoughts . . .
CHERRY PLUM
This remedy is for the feeling of losing control. It is the remedy for those who are afraid their mind might give way, or who are afraid they might do some dreadful thing either to themselves or to someone else. The remedy is also helpful in times of actual loss of control, hysteria, a sudden desire to scream, or for times when we find ourselves in an uncontroll-able rage (so often over something entirely trivial!). This is a wonderful remedy for helping us to put these feelings into place – a remedy for taming the tornado!

For vengeful feelings . . .
HOLLY
This remedy is for feelings of hatred, jealousy, envy, suspi-cion, revenge and is therefore helpful if you should find yourself in a state of spiteful anger, thinking hateful thoughts about another. Holly helps to quash that anger and allow love and compassion to take its place.

For resentment . . .
WILLOW
This remedy is to help any sorrowful feelings that have turned inwards upon oneself – self-pity, resentful introspection, "poor-old-me" etc. For the times when you might be left to do the washing up and, whilst standing at the sink, you begin to resent the fact that it is always down to **you** to do it; resenting your husband for not offering to help; not speaking to him for the rest of the evening, sitting with your arms folded and answering in monosyllables in an attempt to evoke some sympathy . . . We have all felt like this from time to time if we are honest, and during the pre-menstrual phase it is an all too common feeling. The remedy is there, if and when we feel like this, to help us think positively in an outward direction, rather than negatively dwelling inwardly on our misfortune.

For lethargy and procrastination . . .
HORNBEAM
This remedy is for lethargy and weariness; for the feeling of not being "bothered", a desire to cancel the day and return to bed. Hornbeam helps to give us more strength to get on with the day, our work, our life and help us to look forward more optimistically and enthusiastically to what lies ahead.

The cleanser . . .
CRAB APPLE
This is the cleansing remedy, and can be a very helpful complementary remedy to any others that might be needed. The physical bloated feeling, erupting facial blemishes, greasy hair etc., can all create a feeling of ugliness, self-disgust, of being fat and undesirable. As the menses start, some women feel ashamed, unclean, as though some disgusting thing is happening, and that they should wash away their uncleanliness by bathing over and over again. For all these feelings, whether subtle or extreme, Crab Apple is helpful and enables us to appreciate our body and our being for its uniqueness. It helps us to like and love and respect ourselves, to feel proud of who we are, and understand that the menstrual cycle is not a curse or shameful dirty event plaguing us once a month, but instead, a sign of womanhood and wholeness.

CHAPTER THREE

A Question Of Fertility

There are times in most women's lives when, as the months pass, each one marked by the familiar menstrual period, the thought "what is it all about?" creeps into the mind. Perhaps most commonly, this thought would be uppermost in the minds of teenagers because it is then that the term "curse" is really understood! Just at the time when social life is developing and when looks are all important, the appearance of the period can be so distressing. Not only does it bring with it pain and discomfort, but it also causes an increase in the skin's oiliness which in turn frequently causes spots and boils to appear. There can be nothing more frustrating or disheartening than to be looking forward to a special night out when a period starts just at the wrong moment. We learn to live with it as we get a little older, but during the teenage years, it can be catastrophic, especially if that special night out is with a new boyfriend! I do not think there can be many teenage girls who would not welcome some means of abolishing or postponing periods until their purpose is really needed!

For many girls, as relationships with boys begin, and then later on, a more serious relationship with a man develops, the question of sex is bound to arise and needs to be addressed. Most young women are aware and understanding enough to consider this question in a responsible and practical way, but the fear and anxiety attached to the prospect of becoming pregnant or contracting a sexually transmitted disease is very real and something which needs to be thought about carefully. In a woman's younger years, her thoughts tend to be concerned with avoiding pregnancy, and avoiding it at all costs. However, even with the best intentions, theory is inevitably much easier than practice. I can remember, even in my mid-twenties and settled in a secure relationship with my husband, feeling that I would not mind at all if I were rendered sterile – anything to overcome the double headache of avoiding pregnancy and dealing with the nuisance of contraception. Ten years later I realized how naive and shortsighted such ideas were, because the ability to bear a child must be the most precious gift that life has to offer – how ungrateful and selfish to snub it.

During those early years, one can never know how one is going to feel later on, and what life might have in store. We cannot know what we might experience, desire, reject, long for or delight in, and until we do, we can only appreciate how we feel now, and so we act accordingly, without always considering how we **might** feel as a consequence.

FERTILITY

Having had the dangers of taking up a sexual relationship ingrained into us since we were adolescents, many women grow up with the idea that if sexual intercourse takes place, they will, without doubt, become pregnant; a fact of life. However, despite the fact that numerous cases can be cited where a pregnancy has occurred due to an "accident" on the one occasion it took place, there are only a few days in each menstrual cycle during which conception is possible. An ovum can live for only about 24 hours, and although sperm can survive for up to about five days, they need to be in the right place at the right time for fertilization to take place. They need to meet the ovum in the outer segment of the Fallopian tube, which means that intercourse has to take place within about 12 hours of ovulation, or to have taken place in the preceding few days to enable sperm to be in position, ready and waiting for the ovum to be released. Unfortunately, ovulation cannot be predicted accurately enough because although it occurs mid-cycle, it occurs 14 days **before** the onset of menstruation, not 14 days afterwards. If you have a 28 day cycle, then this will in fact be 14 days before **and** afterwards, but if you have a 31 day cycle, ovulation will be 17 days after the onset of your last period, 14 days before the next. Safe practice therefore means using contraceptive measures all the time. Although it is not possible to predict **exactly** when ovulation will take place because the length of our cycle cannot be relied upon no matter how regular it **usually** is (stress and illness for example, can affect the delicate balance of hormones and thus delay ovulation), there are ways and means of establishing that it is about to occur and also when it has actually happened. As the ovum ripens, the cells of the developing follicle produce oestrogen which builds up the endometrium. Oestrogen also causes the cervix to soften or "ripen" and produce a "slippery" mucus. This is called "fertile mucus" as it occurs only during the fertile period of the month. If you make a point of inspecting the mucus produced, you will notice that during the beginning and the end of the cycle, it is opaque and slightly sticky. As mid-cycle approaches, you will notice that it becomes more watery and you will also feel a sensation of "wetness". Then, when ovulation is about to take place, the cervix produces its most fertile mucus which is like the white of an egg, and stretches into a long strand if you hold it between two fingers and slowly draw them apart. Once ovulation has passed, the mucus returns to its usual sticky dryness. The follicle produces progesterone, the hormone that nourishes the ovum and prepares the endometrium for receiving it if it becomes fertilized. Progesterone also causes an increase in the basal body temperature and is in itself, a means of establishing that ovulation has taken place. If the temperature is taken each morning before rising and before eating or drinking, you will notice that after mid-cycle there is a marked increase, and the temperature remains at this higher level until the next period commences when it drops to the lower pre-ovulation level again. Unfortunately, although a fairly accurate diagnosis of ovulation (it is possible to have a temperature rise but not ovulate), it is only useful in retrospect.

HORMONE RELEASE & THEIR EFFECT ON BODY TEMPERATURE AND OVULATION

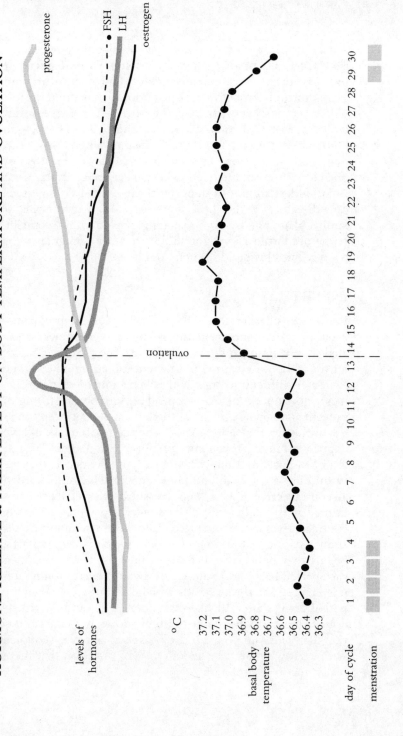

There is, however, a simple test, obtainable from chemists, which will predict when ovulation is about to occur. It measures the levels of Luteinising Hormone in the urine, and as this hormone reaches a peak just prior to ovulation, the test will react positively to this LH surge. A positive result indicates that ovulation will occur during the next 24–36 hours. It is a useful means of coinciding intercourse with ovulation when trying to achieve a pregnancy, but it is not reliable as, nor is it intended to be, a means of contraception.

An understanding of one's fertile and non-fertile periods can, therefore, with a little practice, be used as a means of family planning, by timing intercourse to either coincide with your fertile days if you want to achieve a pregnancy, or by avoiding this period if you do not.

INFERTILITY

Before considering the joys (and anxieties) of pregnancy itself, let us first appreciate the feelings and emotions associated with wanting and trying to have a baby. Some couples hit the jackpot first time, but the emotional traumas can be extremely difficult to cope with when a much wanted pregnancy does not occur. As we spend most of our life trying to prevent a pregnancy by using some form of contraception in the firm belief that a pregnancy is bound to occur should we happen to indulge, even once, in unprotected intercourse, it is a most puzzling thing when we eventually decide that we **would** like a baby, and nothing happens. Having discarded all contraceptive devices, one almost expects to fall pregnant immediately – after all, that is why we were using the contraceptives in the first place! But when each month passes ending with the all too familiar bleeding, it is then that one begins to wonder whether something is wrong, and then each period becomes an anxiously awaited event. If it is late, it is exciting and the heart fills with hope, but then, when the period arrives after all, the disappointment can be tremendous. All those hopes come tumbling down with the realisation that yet again no pregnancy has been achieved, coupled with a growing anxiety and an uneasy suspicion that there really may be a problem.

Anxiety however, can in itself be a fertility antagonist to men and women alike, so worrying whether or not you are fertile may, ironically, be the cause of your infertility. It is a vicious circle and a very difficult one to break. Obviously, something that can relieve the anxiety, depression and strain would help to stop the vicious circle and may be all that is needed to enable the mind and body to relax enough to allow conception to take place. The Bach Remedies, because they are so subtle and benign, are able to gently lift the negative emotions and restore peace and a calmer frame of mind. Remedies need to be selected on an individual basis, but the following list covers the states of mind that are likely to apply.

ASPEN – for the apprehension and anxiety. It is for the strange, uneasy feeling that "something" is about to happen; the remedy for a sense of fear without knowing exactly why you feel afraid, and although in this case the reason for the fear is known, only too well, it is often accompanied by a mixed feeling of uncertain anticipation and anxious excitement. This peculiar sensation can be helped with Aspen.

IMPATIENS – again for anticipation, but this time for impatient anticipation. **WHEN** is it going to happen? Inability to wait; frustration at **having** to wait. Impatience and annoyance when the period arrives, perhaps having a greater impact on those around as we take our frustration out on our nearest and dearest as usual! The Impatiens remedy helps to promote patience and relaxation, so that you are able to take things as they come a little more easily.

WHITE CHESTNUT – the remedy for worrying thoughts that go round and round in the mind allowing no rest and no peace – just a constant bombardment of plans, debates and worries which always seem to be there at the back of the mind, ready to fill the thoughts as soon as there is nothing else to actively occupy the mind at that moment.

GENTIAN – this remedy is for the disappointment, for the set-back and the feeling of having taken two steps forward and one back, or perhaps one forward and two back! This remedy gives encouragement and helps you to take a deep breath and look forward to the next month philosophically and with renewed hope.

There are many other reasons for infertility, or sub-fertility which is, in most cases, a more accurate term, that usually require some form of medical intervention to correct. Admitting that there is a problem is hard enough in itself, but in a way, once this has been overcome and you know that something is going to be done about it, there is a sense of relief as that faint glimmer of hope which had been fading begins to shine more brightly.

Infertility investigations can be lengthy, complex and tedious, and the longer they go on, the heavier the emotional burden becomes, and this goes for both partners. It is a time for sharing and mutual support, and a time when you both need to be strong as you embark upon what might be quite a bumpy ride.

Exactly how lengthy and complex these investigations and subsequent treatment becomes depends on a number of factors. The reasons for the infertility need to be found to begin with, and these may be due to a problem in either the man or the woman, or both. Once the cause has been established treatment can begin, but sometimes the treatment can be far more drawn out and unpredictable than the investigations.

Problems in the man are usually connected with a poor sperm count, and if this is the case, there are some self-help measures which he can take, such as wearing loose trousers, keeping the body cool, taking regular exercise (but avoid strain), reducing alcohol intake and stubbing out the last cigarette once and for all! Sometimes medical treatment may be required to bring the sperm count to a normal level, and if there is a physical problem, corrective medication or surgery may be indicated. Stress in a man however, as mentioned earlier, can also be a major factor when it comes to fertility. Help in this respect to relieve the stress, therefore, will improve the situation, and sometimes this may be all that is required. Often men with responsible or tiring jobs are those who suffer with most stress and tension – men who commute or travel long distances are also often victims of stress. As in all cases, when selecting the most appropriate remedy or remedies, it is essential to consider the individual and choose remedies according to the personality and temperament of the person concerned. Some commonly indicated remedies for men who suffer stress and strain from overwork or tiring jobs are as follows:

VERVAIN – this is the remedy for people who are over-enthusiastic. They enjoy a challenge and take on responsibility as a matter of course. They feel injustice and unfairness strongly and so their enthusiastic nature often drives them to actively protest about a particular issue, or make their opinions known and use their powers of persuasion to win an argument. They tend to overwork, become workaholics and as a result find it hard to switch off and relax. If they have no outlet for their enthusiasm or are unable to channel their ideas, they become frustrated and tense.

ELM – this remedy is for those who are usually capable and confident and have a natural strength to tackle most situations, but at times find that their responsibilities weigh rather heavily, or they feel that they cannot cope when the burden of responsibility placed upon them becomes overwhelming. This is when the Elm person begins to lose confidence and questions whether or not he is as good or capable as he once believed. The Elm remedy therefore helps to restore that faith and confidence.

WHITE CHESTNUT – for mental arguments and agitation – worries about work, money or domestic affairs which can all prey on the mind, and as they do, get out of proportion and begin to dominate the thoughts. A question mark over a man's fertility therefore becomes an additional burden for an already worried and anxious mind, and thus acts as further fuel to generate the circle that is vicious enough already!

AGRIMONY – many men hide the way they feel; they put on a brave face and carefree attitude and appear to take life in their stride – water off a duck's back – whereas in reality, they are secretly worried, afraid, angry or nervous, but do their best to conceal how they really feel. For those of this nature, this remedy is extremely helpful as it soothes the inner turmoil of anguish.

OLIVE – this remedy is for fatigue, and is helpful for those who have a long working day, who work hard and come home feeling exhausted. It is for men who commute and therefore have to leave early and arrive home late, or for those who spend their day travelling – sales representatives or lorry drivers for example. It also helps those involved with a lot of mental work who feel mentally drained.

PINE – this remedy is for feelings of guilt, and it would therefore be helpful for the man who blames himself for his inability to father a child.

Whilst problems in the man seem fairly straightforward and simple to categorize, difficulties in the woman can be much more varied and complex. Reasons for female infertility include:

a) problems with ovulation which may be due to an interference with the release of hormonal messages, or the reception of those messages by the ovary, or due to ovarian disease;

b) difficulties in connection with the journey from the ovary to uterus which could be due to damaged Fallopian tubes, perhaps as a result of pelvic infection or complications after surgery;

c) difficulties in connection with the uterus itself – the lining may not be sufficiently receptive or there may be an obstruction such as a fibroid or polyp.

d) Other factors such as endocrine disorders affecting organs, e.g. the thyroid gland, which in turn affect the reproductive cycle indirectly, or physical abnormalities such as missing or malformed organs.

There are numerous reasons, and considering the delicate balance and complex workings of the female reproductive system, it is not surprising that there are so many things that can potentially go wrong.

The normal recommendation is that help should be sought if the couple have tried unsuccessfully to have a baby for about a year. Some doctors will instigate infertility investigations only after two years of trying, others will intervene after about six months. Generally, it depends on age – the older you are, the sooner investigations should begin because after the age of about 25 a woman's natural fertility is already beginning to decline! However, many couples now choose to wait until the age of about thirty or thirty plus before deciding to start a family, giving the woman a chance to pursue her own career and ambitions. Unfortunately it also means that if she does experience difficulties in becoming pregnant, time is no longer on her side. Alas, there is no way of knowing beforehand.

Medical Intervention – a typical programme

Having recognized that there is a problem and sought medical help, both partners will need to be examined and undergo some preliminary tests. These include a semen analysis and sperm count for the man, and various blood tests for the woman to determine the hormone levels and thus identify where the problem might lie. Quite often, the woman will also need to undergo a small operation to eliminate any physical abnormality or dysfunction. This operation is called a 'laparoscopy' and usually involves an overnight stay in hospital. The surgeon makes a tiny incision in the abdomen and inserts an instrument which allows him to see clearly the state of the ovaries, uterus and Fallopian tubes. If there is a problem he will be able to recommend appropriate treatment or may be able to correct the problem there and then. Laparoscopy itself is quite a painless operation and causes very little discomfort. It does, however, involve filling the abdomen with gas so that the organs are easily visible, so a common post-operative complaint is 'wind' which seems to be "locked in" and can be quite painful. The best way to overcome it is to move about – get up and walk around to give it a chance to dissipate, which brings great relief.

The prospect of any operation is daunting, and some people find it much more frightening than others – or perhaps some people admit to being afraid more than others! Either way, the Remedies can help to calm the mind before and afterwards. **RESCUE REMEDY** particularly is a helpful stand-by and will ease the panic and fear of what is to come, as well as easing the trauma of the ordeal itself. By aiding our whole system emotionally in this way, the body will be able to begin its own healing straight away. **MIMULUS** is also helpful at this time, being the remedy for known fears, and so if you are afraid or nervous about what might happen, the results or the pain, Mimulus will help ease that nervousness. Coupled with known fears are those of a vague and unknown nature – apprehension and unexplained panic. These feelings are helped by the remedy **ASPEN**. For worrying thoughts, perhaps causing sleeplessness, **WHITE CHESTNUT** is helpful. Post-operatively, if you should feel depressed for no apparent reason – for example, if the operation went well and revealed no abnormalities, yet you feel low instead of being filled with relief and restored hope, then **MUSTARD** is the remedy you need to help that dark cloud move away. If however, some abnormality **is** found and the news causes you to feel disheartneed and the reason for the depression is therefore known, **GENTIAN** is the remedy to lift your spirits and give you the encouragement you need to look ahead more positively.

Having either corrected the problem found during laparoscopy, or having established that no physical abnormalities exist, the next stage will be to look more closely, if necessary, at the sequence of events that should result in successful ovulation. A hormonal problem responsible for inefficiencies in this area is usually detected through blood tests, but inactive ovaries can also be detected visually during laparoscopy. Either way, the usual first line treatment is with a drug called Clomiphene. This drug reduces the level of oestrogen in the system thereby stimulating a lazy pituitary gland to increase its production of Follicle Stimulating Hormone. Clomiphene is regarded as a very successful fertility drug, resulting in pregnancy in about 65% of women treated, although it still may take a little while. A normally fertile couple would not expect to conceive immediately – within about 6 months is average – so do not be too disheartened if the treatment does not achieve a pregnancy straight away. If

Clomiphene does not produce the desired results after a reasonable length of time, the next step is to try giving Follicle Stimulating Hormone (FSH) itself, and thus rather than rely on the pituitary to produce a sufficient amount in response to the action of Clomiphene, the hormone is given directly by injection. The drug used for this purpose is known as Human Menopausal Gonadotrophin (HMG) and is prepared, as the name suggests, from the urine of menopausal women whose pituitary glands produce large quantities of FSH in an attempt to stimulate ovarian function. One of the most favoured brands of HMG is Pergonal. Treatment with Pergonal often succeeds where Clomiphene fails but it is a much more involved programme requiring careful monitoring to reduce the risks of over-stimulation of the ovaries. Under this treatment, there is a distinct possibility and increased incidence of multiple birth as more than one follicle frequently develops to maturity. It is, however, a risk that most women find well worth taking, but hyperstimulation can result in cyst formation which is why a close eye is kept on developments at the appropriate times. A typical treatment regime would include a series of injections early in the cycle, followed by an ultrasound scan of the ovaries in mid-cycle to check progress. When a follicle or follicles are ripe, an injection of Human Chorionic Gonadotrophin (a pregnancy hormone that has the same effect as Luteinizing Hormone) is given to stimulate ovulation. A smaller dose is repeated about a week later to encourage implantation. Some women may require a combination of both Clomiphene and Pergonal to obtain optimum follicle development.

A treatment programme such as this requires a great deal of stamina. It can be tiring, inconvenient and demoralizing. It is, however, an **active** treatment and so at least you know what is happening – you know whether the ovum is ripening, when it is ripe and when it is being released. This knowledge is reassuring because it gives hope in there being a real chance that a pregnancy may be achieved. It also provides sound information about the most fertile time of the month and thus the optimum time for intercourse. It does however, have a distinct drawback – it makes it all so pre-meditated and clinical, that sex may then become just a baby-making process instead of the tender and spontaneous expression of love between a man and a woman. As time goes on, ensuring that it takes place on the right day can become an obsession, and love-making is then soon in danger of becoming a calendar event, booked in advance – "tonight's the night" whether you feel like it or not! Most doctors will also request that a temperature chart is kept. This is an interesting and very useful way of gaining an insight into what is happening, but it is another burden; something else to worry about, something else to be dictated by. If you are not careful, the calendar or temperature chart may soon be ruling your entire life!

> "Weary with toil, I haste me to my bed,
> The dear repose for limbs with travel tired;
> But then begins a journey in my head,
> To work my mind, when body's work's expired:
> For then my thoughts, from far where I abide,
> Intend a zealous pilgrimage to thee,
> And keep my drooping eyelids open wide,
> Looking on darkness which the blind do see:
> Save that my soul's imaginary sight
> Presents thy shadow to my sightless view,
> Which, like a jewel hung in ghastly night,
> Makes black night beauteous, and her old face new,
> Lo, thus, by day my limbs, by night my mind,
> For thee, and for myself, no quiet find."

> William Shakespeare

Always an 'Auntie', never a mother. . . .
The whole business can become a complete obsession. It is a time for sharing, and if you CAN help each other through it, then the journey will be that much easier. There is a lot of truth in the old saying "a problem shared is a problem halved" – it may not be halved exactly, but at least the heavy burden can be shared and not borne by one alone. Unfortunately the emotional anguish, confusion and uncertainty is something that is difficult to put into words, or the right words, and consequently often goes unmentioned. For both

partners it is a difficult time, but for the woman it can be unbearable. Her natural maternal instincts and desire to not only have a baby and raise a child but to actually **carry** it; experience motherhood in its entirety which includes the pregnancy itself, is very strong. Getting pregnant and being pregnant therefore soon becomes the first line ambition – motherhood itself drifts into the distance and almost becomes an added bonus to the fulfilment and satisfaction of achieving the primary objective. This is where a woman obsessed can easily become a woman possessed as she finds herself spending more and more time in the library or book shop, scanning the shelves for a book that just **might** contain the answers to all her problems. Sadly, the more she reads, the more depressing the whole situation becomes. Statistics, percentages and graphs do not offer much hope, and ultimately, having read virtually every book written on the subject of infertility, she is left with all the uncertainty and frustration she had in the first place, and often a lot more, as she looks ahead to an even bleaker vision of the future than she may have ever imagined!

There are however, always sparks of hope, when a period is late and the inevitable thought enters the mind, "perhaps, just **perhaps**, I might be . . . " but quickly put out of the mind again for fear of tempting fate! All too often "fate" is a bit *too* quick off the mark, and snatches that glimmer of hope away before it has even had a chance to become a serious consideration. In the meantime, however, during those few fretful days waiting and wondering, every little sign, every little symptom becomes a major focal point – "I think I felt sick; was that a tingle I felt in my breast?; I've gone off coffee – I MUST be pregnant!" And then, for a fleeting moment, you allow yourself to feel just a tiny bit excited, and then find yourself back in the book-shop again, this time looking for books to confirm that you **are** pregnant, a chapter that will list in graphic detail **every single** conceivable symptom about how you should feel, something to identify with, latch onto and anticipate.

The drop back into reality when the appearance of menstruation signals all too clearly the end of all those hopes and dreams, is a very sharp and hard drop indeed – back to earth with a bump to put it mildly! Despair, anguish, heartache, anger, misery, all set in again. Even when you try to get away from it by losing yourself in something else – shopping, watching television, going for a drive – there is "always something there to remind you". The shops seem to be full of childrens' clothes, toys or pregnant women! Television programmes all seem to relate to babies in some way. Even the sight of a car with the announcement "baby on board" displayed in the back window by the proud parents, is like a clanging of bells mocking "we've got a baby and you haven't". You know it is irrational to think this way, but you cannot help it. And no matter how trivial it may seem, how you long to hang a similar sign in the back of YOUR car.

It can seem a very sad and unfair fact of life that pregnancy is something the average woman spends her entire reproductive life either trying to avoid or achieve. Some people find it hard to avoid, others find it hard to achieve, and whichever it is, not everyone is happy with the result. Some who fall pregnant easily are those who would most prefer *not* to, and by the same token, those who find it hard to achieve a pregnancy are often those who long for a baby the most. Life certainly is not always easy, and things do not always happen the way we would like them to. There are, however, lessons to be learned from every experience in life and sometimes the biggest and hardest lesson of all is ACCEPTANCE. Acceptance of something the way it is, and acceptance of the fact that what we want is not always what we get! Coming to terms with childlessness when you so desperately want a baby has to be one of the most difficult hurdles life has to offer. To approach it philosophically and ACCEPT it as a way of life takes incalculable courage and strength. Acceptance is, essentially, a demonstration of one's faith in life itself because absolute acceptance is absolute faith – trust and belief in one's own destiny. It is a hard thing to come to terms with, and most people grapple with it for years, but that is NORMAL. It is human nature, and because we are human beings, it is natural for us to struggle on, try anything, go to all lengths to fight for what we want, try and MAKE life go the way we want it. But of course we cannot force it, and by attempting to do so we work ourselves up into a state of high tension, unable to relax or think of anything else. Ironically, this dreadful anguish can be the very thing standing in the way of success, and yet it can be so difficult to be consistently positive in outlook; to give the body a chance to actually respond. It just becomes a vicious circle. Nothing happens because you are so uptight, and you are so uptight because nothing happens! Quite often it is when a woman finally gives up and resigns herself to childlessness that conception occurs – due to a relaxation of mental tension. The balance between mind and body is so fine that prolonged anxiousness at a time like this can have the most dramatic effect on the body, and so it is most important to maintain a calm and positive outlook, to be happy and relaxed, and to think philosphically and positively about the realities that might have to be endured. Easier said than done, perhaps, but that is what the Remedies are there for – to help us to achieve that inner peace and give us the strength to face up to one of the hardest experiences of life. Some that are particularly useful to consider are as follows:

SWEET CHESTNUT – for the despair; the feeling that there is no end in sight, for absolute helplessness, knowing there is nothing you can do and for the awful heartache that fills the soul when another month comes to an end and another period begins. It is the sort of feeling that is there deep inside, with you when you wake up and with you when you go to bed, perhaps momentarily relieved during the fleeting moments during arousal from sleep until your conscious mind reminds you of your grief. This remedy is wonderful should you ever feel like this. It gently lifts that awful despair and replaces it with an enriched sense of security, with happier thoughts, a hopeful approach and a reassuring embrace that all will be well.

HOLLY – for the anger and jealousy that may be aroused.

HEATHER – for those who are obsessed with their troubles and difficulties, thinking about nothing else and taking the opportunity to talk about them to others when the chance arises, disinterested in any other topic of conversation. Heather will help to take your mind off yourself and to be able to think and communicate more openly, free from the constraints of self absorption.

CHERRY PLUM – for the uncontrollable irrational thoughts, when the imagination runs riot.

STAR OF BETHLEHEM – for the sense of loss; the grief associated with the child you do not have but desperately want; the sadness and emptiness that fills the heart as each potentially hopeful month comes to an end.

GENTIAN – for the disappointment and despondency that is caused by either the infertility itself or the treatment programme you may have to undergo.

GORSE – for loss of hope; for a pessimistic outlook, feeling as though there is no point in proceeding as you will never achieve success. Gorse, if you feel like this, will help you to regain that hope so that you can look forward with more optimism.

WILLOW – for resentment and bitterness towards life, or towards other women who do not seem to be burdened with such misfortune. This feeling can be difficult to shake off and may soon start to eat away at your happiness and ability to enjoy life. It begins to draw you down like a whirlpool, your thoughts becoming more and more introspective causing a miserable depression. The Willow remedy helps you to resist the whirlpool effect and be able to cast your mind outward to see the good things in life, not only the bad.

WHITE CHESTNUT – this remedy will complement the others, helping to settle your thoughts and allowing your mind to relax. It is a great relief to be able to "switch off" the constant mental chatter, just as though you had turned off an annoying record that had stuck in the groove; you don't always notice how annoying it was until peace and quiet is restored!

Desperately wanting a baby, trying so hard and for so long, generates all kinds of feelings and stirs emotions you never thought you had. Everything is exaggerated the longer time goes on, and when you see what seems like **everyone** else producing children as though it were as easy as shelling peas, life can seem terribly unfair. It seems as though you are the only one who has difficulty (**WILLOW**). Indeed it should be the easiest thing in the world to make a baby – after all, that is what we are designed for. What could be more natural? What could be simpler? Why then, is nothing happening? This frustration and sense of injustice that leads to tension and exasperation is helped enormously with the remedy **VERVAIN**. A woman in this kind of emotional trauma can feel so isolated and lonely, and the loneliness is worsened by her own reluctance to disclose her true feelings to others (**AGRIMONY**), and her reluctance to admit totally, even to herself, that there really is a problem. It is as though by keeping quiet the problem will automatically resolve itself, and by burying her head in the sand the whole thing will somehow be easier to bear. The Bach Remedies play an important role in our emotional health and stability, but as well as taking a selection of remedies to help the way you feel, it can be helpful to talk to a counsellor – either a Counsellor in the Bach Flower Remedies (the Bach Centre keeps a register of trained practitioners) to help with your choice, or as a therapeutic aid in itself. It can certainly be helpful to open up to **someone**, particularly if it is someone who has experienced or is experiencing similar difficulties as it instils hope and gives encouragement, and reinstates faith in achieving your goal. It also helps to know that you are **not** the only one. In fact, infertility is much more common than most people believe to be the case. It is reported that about 1 in 15 couples experience difficulty conceiving. There are a number of support groups which offer help, guidance and mutual support through their membership, and so it may be worthwhile considering approaching one of those. Sharing your problem with others who are in the same boat can, for some, be extremely therapeutic, and releasing all those feelings that you have not confronted before can be an enormous relief.

Helping yourself naturally

There are also other very simple and practical measures that can be taken to maximise your chances. These are basically centered around keeping healthy and fit. A good diet containing all the necessary trace elements and vitamins, such as Zinc and Magnesium, both found in wheat germ, Iodine found in sea-food, and the B-Complex vitamins found in green vegetables, wholegrains, nuts, milk, eggs, pulses and brewer's yeast are all necessary for normal fertility, and so it would be wise to make sure that your diet provides all these vital ingredients. In addition to this, try to eliminate ingredients which are or may potentially be, a hindrance to fertility or may prevent the vital substances from working efficiently or being adequately absorbed into the system – coffee; alcohol; nicotine for example. Also, check your weight – if you are OVER weight or UNDER weight, this may be a contributing factor and so would be wise to correct. However, if you need to lose weight, do it gradually, and do not deprive yourself of any necessary daily nutritional requirements as this would be counter-productive. Weight loss should at the best of times be gradual, because it is healthier and more effective, but it is particularly important to lose excess weight slowly when you are hoping to become pregnant because rapid weight loss causes the body to break down fat swiftly to provide sufficient energy. This fat breakdown causes an increase in a substance called KETONES in the blood, and it is possible that high levels of this, such as may occur on a very strict fast weight loss programme, may be potentially harmful to a developing foetus. As you will not **know** that you are pregnant until at least 2 weeks after conception, it makes sense to be prepared, and lose weight slowly, just in case! Alternatively, make a point of losing weight first, and put your attempts at conception on hold for a couple of months or so. The advantage is that during this time you will also have a chance to take regular exercise – nothing too energetic or strenuous, but something that will gently enhance your general well-being, such as walking, swimming, cycling, yoga or "Swing-into-Shape". Exercise is extremely therapeutic so it is a good idea to take it up and make it routine whether you are trying to lose weight or not. It increases the circulating oxygen in the blood, so it is even better if your exercise, or some of it, is taken out of doors; it reduces fatigue and energizes stagnant muscle tissue. It also increases the metabolism so you feel less lethargic and altogether brighter. This in turn naturally helps your emotional outlook as it increases the oxygen supply to the brain (as well as every-where else which, of course, includes the reproductive organs!) and thus helps you feel more positive and "alive".

Your partner too can take some simple measures to opti-mize his fertility. Sperm do not develop or survive in condi-tions that are too warm, which is why a man's testicles are outside the body. Thus, to wear trousers or underpants that are too tight, will make the testes too warm and inhibit healthy sperm production. It is therefore preferable to wear boxer shorts as these are cooler, and conventional trousers as they are looser and provide more freedom, fashionable or not! If he can bear it, he might also take a cold shower each day – not much fun in the winter months, but it does help to keep the scrotum cool nevertheless! And he too should lose excess weight, take regular exercise, reduce alcohol and coffee consumption if excessive, and avoid tobacco altogether as this has a well-known dampening effect on sperm production.

There are also some therapeutic aids that you may like to pursue to increase your natural fertility. Acupuncture, chi-ropractic, reflexology and aromatherapy can all stimulate the reproductive organs, their nerve impulses or blood supply, and if your problem is due to an "energy block" in this sense, then one of these therapies may provide your answer. You may also find benefit through spiritual healing. Meditation helps to unclutter the mind, clear it of the thoughts that buzz around all day, and helps you to train your thoughts to focus on positive things and draw positive energy into your sys-tem. The Bach Remedies will help to ease a troubled mind, but you can help the whole process along by actively doing something to encourage positive thought. Meditation com-bined with yoga has wonderfully energizing and relaxing benefits. It is not everybody's cup of tea, and indeed some people find it too difficult to relax enough to accomplish it successfully, but I **would** recommend that you try. It is both calming and enlivening, and **very** therapeutic.

CHAPTER FOUR

Pregnancy And Childbirth

The controversy over exactly when a new human life begins is considerable. Some consider it to be the moment when the sperm and ovum unite; other schools of thought would say it does not begin until the fertilized ovum implants itself in the uterus; some do not consider the developing embryo to be "alive" until it is actually capable of independent survival at about 28 weeks gestation. It is the question mark over precisely when human life begins that is central to the arguments surrounding abortion, which is of course a controversial issue in itself, and something we will consider in a little more detail in the next chapter.

In the meantime, let's have a look at the actual sequence of events that lead up to conception and how the baby develops. We have already seen how, during the menstrual cycle, the ovum matures and is released from the ovary with its hopes held high of meeting a strong and healthy sperm on its way along the Fallopian tube. We also know that intercourse must take place during the fertile period of the cycle, that is, around the time of ovulation. Preferably, this would be just before ovulation when the conditions are at their best – when the cervical mucus is easily penetrable by sperm and is at its most "nutritious" (it nourishes the sperm during the first part of their journey), when the uterine lining is most receptive and when the ovum is about to be released. The sperm deposited at the cervix during intercourse begin to swim upwards through the cervical canal, into the uterus itself and then along the Fallopian tube. It is quite a long and arduous journey and only the strongest will actually make it. Some will have perished before even reaching the cervical canal, others will perish on their way through the main body of the uterus, others will head for the wrong tube. Approximately 200 million sperm are produced in each ejaculation, and yet only about 100 actually reach the ovum. It is, therefore, just as well that a man produces so many each time!

The Fallopian tube is lined with microscopic hairs called cilia. The cilia, together with the muscular contractions along the length of Fallopian tube, propel the ovum towards the uterus. The sperm, therefore, have to swim against the tide – another test of their endurance! As they meet, the sperm that are still viable connect with the ovum and attach themselves to its outer coat. Now begins the final race. As they all begin to 'feed', and digest the outer coating of the ovum; only one will actually penetrate its shell. That one sperm, having made its way inside, fuses with the nucleus of the ovum and produces a substance which kills the other contenders. It is then that fertilization has taken place. The fertilized ovum continues its journey along the remaining length of the Fallopian tube and the cells rapidly begin dividing. Soon, a small cystic structure known as a "blastocyst" is formed. It is at this stage of development that the uterine cavity is reached, four days after fertilization. The blatocyst settles on the uterine lining and its cells begin to digest the surface as it embeds itself. This is when conception is said to have occurred. It continues to bury itself deeper and deeper into the endometrium (now called "decidua" – the term for a "pregnant endometrium") until it is completely concealed, about 13 days after ovulation. This is the time when the menstrual period would normally be due, but if conception has taken place, that period will not materialize. A missed period is probably the most obvious sign of pregnancy and is certainly the most likely cause of amenorrhoea in a healthy woman of childbearing age who has had normal and regular previous cycles. It is, however, one of the most frequently missed signs, and is often only noticed in hindsight, because unless a woman is particularly concerned about her fertility or is using fertile signs as a means of contraception, she may not keep anything other than a rough mental note of when her period is due, and may not notice at all until it is a week or two late. By that time, other signs and symptoms will probably be alerting her to the possibility or probability of a developing pregnancy.

As the blastocyst develops, its cells become differentiated. The outer cells continue to grow and eventually become the placenta, completely formed by 13 weeks. The inner cells form the gestational sac and the embryo. The developing pregnancy, until the placenta takes over, is nourished by progesterone and oestrogen produced by the corpus luteum, the "yellow body" that filled the empty follicle in the ovary after ovulation (see Chapter Two). In a normal non-pregnant cycle, corpus luteum develops and produces progesterone which is the hormone responsible for most of the pre-menstrual symptoms. In pregnancy the production of both hormones increase and their combined symptomatic effect is that much greater, giving rise to the classic pregnancy symptoms such as nausea, the urge to pass urine more frequently and tingling, tender, swollen breasts. Progesterone is also responsible for the formation of the decidua. Oestrogen is responsible for growth, and both hormones play a part in the development of the milk producing system of the breasts.

Without a doubt, the surge of hormones during pregnancy is responsible for a variety of emotional ups and downs as well as physical symptoms and disturbances. But super-imposed upon the hormone-related upsets are the normal, natural emotions that would be felt and experienced regard-less of how much or how little progesterone is circulating in the body! That is, feeling elated or depressed **because** you are pregnant rather than **due to** the pregnancy itself.

If you have planned to have a baby or perhaps not actually planned it, but found the discovery a happy surprise, or you have been trying unsuccessfully for some time, the realization that you have a baby developing inside you will fill you with delight. Filled with joy, you will be unlikely to need any remedies at this stage – they are for negative emotions, and you could not feel more positive! However, this intitial elation may be dampened a little once the idea has had a chance to sink in, with anxieties, fears and doubts about your ability to cope with the responsibility of bringing a new human being into the world. The Remedies can therefore be of help right from the start, enabling you to put those niggling doubts and fears into perspective before they have a chance to grow out of proportion and spoil what should otherwise be nine months of happy fulfilment.

MIMULUS is the rememdy if you feel afraid – afraid of the birth, or pain, afraid of complications, or of there being something wrong with the baby.

ASPEN is the remedy for the sort of fear that is less definable – a strange sense of apprehension, foreboding, fear of the unknown.

ELM if you feel doubtful about your ability to cope, feeling suddenly overwhelmed with responsibility.

MUSTARD for an unexplained depression. You know you should be happy – after all, this is what you wanted – but feel so low in your spirits you cannot be at all joyful. It is as though a heavy dark cloud has descended on your life, but you do not know why and are powerless to cast it aside.

WALNUT for the changes going on within you – your body is going through a tremendous period of adjustment and it is because it is unsettling that the hormones are having such an impact on you. Walnut is the remedy to even out the humps and bumps to give you a smoother ride.

CHERRY PLUM if you feel you are losing control. This feeling can be very frightening, and it can help to understand **why** you might feel like this, i.e. to understand the imbalance caused by the surge of hormonal activity as well as the physical changes taking place so quickly – a combination of all these things may make you feel that you are losing control of your rational senses, and if you should experience such emotions, this remedy will help you to regain your sanity.

STAR OF BETHLEHEM for the shock to the system. It may have felt rather like a dream, but all of a sudden, the reality of the pregnancy hits you, and Star of Bethlehem is the remedy to buffer the shock.

CLEMATIS – this is for dreaminess, the far-away sensation as though life is going on around you, but you are somehow removed from it. Not a panicky feeling – that would be **ROCK ROSE** – but rather a stunned, bemused feeling, or one of mental escapism and fantasy. Clematis is the remedy to help you gather your thoughts from orbit and bring them back to earth into the here and now.

We have concentrated so far, on how delightful pregnancy can be, and on women who set out happily to start a family. There are, however, some women who do not want children. Finding out you are pregnant, therefore, may not be such a happy occasion. It may indeed be the very **last** thing you wanted. It may spell disaster for one reason or another; something you have always dreaded. And so, what in some women generates a bouncing mood, can be for others, quite depressing. It is then that negative feelings come to the fore, yet they are often replaced by more positive thoughts once the idea has had a chance to settle and you have come to terms with the fact that your plans may have to CHANGE but do not necessarily need to come to an end! In the meantime, however, there are a number of remedies which can help, depending on how it has affected you personally.

STAR OF BETHLEHEM for the shock.

WALNUT to help you adjust.

HOLLY for the vengeful feelings.

ROCK ROSE for terror or panic.

WILLOW for resentment or bitterness.

CHICORY for selfishness.

CRAB APPLE for self-disgust, self-hatred, feeling contaminated; a desire to get rid of the "parasite" inside you. This remedy also helps if you feel ashamed of your pregnant state, the sight of your growing body; feeling embarrased by it.

ROCK WATER if you find you are severely reprimanding yourself for "being so stupid", feeling that you have let yourself down.

PINE if you feel you have let others down, or feel guilty.

SWEET CHESTNUT for a feeling of despair, feeling ensnared; trapped, with no way of escape.

As the pregnancy develops, your own body is in effect playing host to the baby which feeds off your resources. Whilst you do not need to "eat for two", you will need to make sure that you are taking a balanced and nutritious diet containing all the necessary vitamins, minerals, protein and fibre in all the right quantities so that your own system can remain in healthy working order. The foetus will take its nourishment first and deplete your store cupboard if you are not taking a sufficient amount. So, as the Boy Scouts would say, "be prepared", and make sure that your intake provides enough for both your needs. This does not mean over-eating – a normal diet should provide all the nutrients required for both mother and baby, but there are certain trace elements that are required in greater quantities, so your diet needs to be rich in certain foods to cater for these demands.

You will put on about 12.5 kilos in weight (about 2 stone) during the course of your pregnancy. A small proportion of this is extra fat, but thankfully, most of it is due to the pregnancy itself and will therefore be shed when the baby is born. The following breakdown shows how that 12.5 kg is accounted for:

Foetus	3.4 kg
Placenta	0.6 kg
Amniotic fluid	0.8 kg
Increased weight of uterus	0.9 kg
Increased weight of breasts	0.4 kg
Increase in blood volume	1.5 kg
Extra-cellular fluid	1.4 kg
Fat	3.4 kg
Total	12.5 kg

Your pregnancy should develop healthily without you putting on any **excess** weight – that is fat unrelated to the pregnancy itself which will not disappear when the baby is born. It is natural for pregnant women to feel hungry at certain stages of their pregnancy, and this is nature's way of indicating that further nutritional supplies are needed. If you receive these signals, try to avoid **fattening** foods in-between meals – opt for a piece of fruit or something that will actually have the dual purpose of satisfying your hunger as well as providing some healthy nutrients, rather than just loading your system with extra calories! Some women however, develop cravings for certain foods – cream cakes or chocolate biscuits for example. Although it is important to be sensible about what you eat, it is not necessary to become a **"ROCK WATER"** over it – intransigent and self sacrificing! Enjoy the odd nicety, treat yourself now and then to something you fancy – just don't overdo it! And indeed, those cravings, like the hunger pangs, may just be nature's way of telling you what your body needs – well, even if it is not, it's a comforting thought!

THE FIRST TRIMESTER

During the early stages of pregnancy, changes in appetite are probably the most noticeable. Nausea and vomiting, although notoriously in the early morning, and among the first and most classic of all pregnancy symptoms, can occur at any time of the day, but thankfully this rather unpleasant symptom is relatively short lasting, and generally ceases to be a problem after about 16 weeks. **CRAB APPLE** although not a remedy for sickness as such, may, as it is the cleansing remedy, help you feel a little better during this period. **RESCUE REMEDY** too may also be helpful. Running parallel to the nausea, some women have an aversion to certain foods – "going off" coffee for example, or finding the smell of cigarette smoke intolerable. Just as some cravings may be nature's way of letting you know that your body needs certain foods, so this too is nature's way of protecting the pregnancy from the potentially harmful effects of certain foodstuffs or substances. There are, however, in contrast, many women who are not affected by these palatal changes and so do not need to alter their eating habits. Similarly, some women who smoke continue to do so throughout their pregnancy. This does not, however, suggest that because there is no apparent aversion to it, that it will not do any harm. The dangers of smoking are well known and well documented. It pregnancy it not only destroys certain vitamins and trace elements and depletes the body's natural ability to absorb vital nutrients, but also affects the health of the placenta, causing it to be smaller and prone to infarction, when a small area or areas die. As the placenta is the baby's source of nutrition and oxygen, the health of the baby is directly dependent on the health of the placenta. If it is unhealthy, there is an obvious risk to the unborn infant.

There are, however, other noxious substances, besides nicotine, that can also penetrate the placental barrier (rather like a sieve; some substances pass through whilst others do not) – some drugs, prescribed and over-the-counter – Aspirin for example, and some antibiotics, as well as "social" drugs and alcohol, all pass through the placental membrane and enter the baby's blood stream which is, apart from this placental link, entirely independent of your own.

As the level of the hormone progesterone rises, it has a relaxing effect on the smooth involuntary muscle and this causes the muscles in the gut to relax which can give rise to constipation, and relaxation of the muscles surrounding the bladder and urethra causing disturbances in micturition. The pressure of the growing pregnancy on the bladder is, however, also partially responsible for this. Progesterone also relaxes the muscular walls of the blood vessels which is why the blood pressure tends to drop in pregnancy, although other, rather less common complications, may cause it to be raised.

With all these changes going on within your body, it is no wonder that tiredness is another common symptom! Actually some women experience a strange sense of fatigue very early on in pregnancy, even before the first period has been missed, but as the pregnancy develops and the baby is growing, the physical effort involved in carrying all those extra pounds around all day, every day, can become a strain, gradually sapping your energy – like picking up a heavy shopping bag that you know you will not be able to put down again for the next nine months! The remedy to help ease the fatigue is **OLIVE** – wonderfully restorative for this kind of tiredness. Add two drops to a glass of water, or make up a treatment bottle if you are going out, and take regular and frequent doses until you are feeling better.

Other remedies which can play an important and helpful role are:

WALNUT for the series of changes that your whole system needs to rapidly and constantly adjust to;

PINE if you feel guilty or blame yourself – perhaps believing that you have harmed your baby in some way and cannot free your mind from the thought;

CRAB APPLE has already been mentioned with regard to nausea, but it is a helpful remedy whenever you feel the need for a cleanser, even if it is because you don't like to look at yourself, or just have a general feeling of unpleasantness;

MIMULUS is the remedy should you feel afraid – perhaps of something going wrong with the pregnancy or with the baby's development;

RED CHESTNUT if the fears are out of proportion and are centred around the baby's well-being, becoming over-concerned and anxious about its health and safety, perhaps to the extent that you are afraid to walk to the shops, take a bath or empty your bowels in case it will damage the baby in some way. These fears will be heightened if you have experienced a miscarriage in the past, because you will naturally be more protective and careful about everything you do.

Colds and other viruses can also be a worry. Indeed, you should seek advice if you become unwell so that your own health as well as that of the baby can be monitored a little more closely. Generally, common colds run their course and do not present any great problems – more of an inconvenience than anything else – but some other infections might be harmful if left unchecked, so it is always best to seek medical advice and nip it in the bud before it gets any worse. **CRAB APPLE** however, is a helpful remedy to take at this time to aid the body's natural ability to cleanse itself, and **OLIVE** and **HORNBEAM** for the fatigue and weariness associated with most depressions in health. Other remedies too, given in accordance with your general outlook and personality type will help you to fight illness.

Stress, strain, worry, anxiousness etc., all disrupt body chemistry and throw the system out of balance. It is then that our natural resources which are otherwise very capable of withstanding ill health, become low, and when depleted in this way, the door is open to the invasion of disease. It therefore follows that to tackle the stress, worry, fear etc., **before** it has such devastating effects on our natural strength, will maintain optimum health and well-being. This is especially important during pregnancy because heavy emotional disturbances can disrupt its development and affect the pregnancy as much as the physical impact of disease and the substances previously mentioned. The Bach Flower Remedies are a very gentle system of helping us to achieve and maintain that inner emotional balance, thus giving ourselves the chance to enjoy a healthy and stress-free pregnancy, and for the unborn baby, a peaceful introduction to its first nine months of life.

THE SECOND TRIMESTER

The middle three months of pregnancy are usually the most enjoyable. The unpleasant symptoms of early pregnancy are over and the final stages and the birth itself are far enough away not to present any difficulties. This is the time to really enjoy it, and get used to the idea of being a mother. Somewhere between about 16 and 20 weeks of gestation, you will begin to feel the baby moving inside you – "foetal movements". These are rather like a fluttering inside the abdomen and could be mistaken for pockets of moving wind! Women who have been pregnant before often notice these movements earlier – around 16 weeks just when the baby is mature enough to make an impact – because they recognize the familiar feeling. First time mothers do not usually notice foetal movements until about 20 weeks when they are rather more unmistakable. The experience of your baby moving inside you is the first really positive sign that there **really is** a baby – it's true, not just a dream! – and it is this knowledge that brings about a warmness, the first stages of bonding, towards your unborn child. As the weeks pass, this warmness develops and becomes deeper. You become more aware of the baby's presence, you feel more protective; more of a mother. This mid-trimester is therefore an exciting time and it is little wonder that women at this stage of pregnancy seem to be in full bloom, radiating a healthy glow all around them.

This is also the time when your instinct for "nest-building" begins – when you seem to find a burst of energy to spring-clean the house, or re-decorate – something you may have been putting off for months! You will also find yourself, if you have not done so already, looking at baby clothes, cots, prams, child safety seats and, at long last, those "baby on board" window stickers! It may seem strange to feel so emotional about such everyday things, but if you have waited a long time for this moment to arrive, then you deserve to indulge yourself – so go on, enjoy it!

THE THIRD TRIMESTER

During the final three months, from about 24 weeks onwards, the pregnancy develops noticeably at a very rapid
rate. All the organs, limbs and extremities will have already
developed and so this period is the one devoted mainly to
growth. The pregnancy becomes heavy towards the end, and
this in itself may cause some discomfort such as backache,
odd nerve pains as the baby lies in an uncomfortable position,
additional tiredness, and heartburn due to the pressure of the
baby on the stomach as well as to the action of progesterone,
relaxing the sphincter muscle at the entrance to the stomach
which normally prevents stomach juices spilling back into
the oesophagus or gullet. At about 36 weeks, the baby has
turned itself upside down and begins to descend head-first
into the cavity of the pelvis. The pelvis is capable of containing the entire head and once it has done so, it is said to be
"engaged". Understandably, the familiar symptom associated with early pregnancy – frequent desire to pass water –
returns, but this time, due to the pressure of the baby's head
on the bladder! At about this stage of pregnancy, the end is
clearly in sight, and you may begin to feel a little impatient,
wishing the time away to the expected date of delivery. Your
impatience with time may also make you a little impatient
with other people, and in particular your partner or someone
else close to you – the same people who receive the brunt of
those pre-menstrual tensions and frustrations! **IMPA-
TIENS** is the remedy to help you to relax during these last
days or weeks, and help you to settle instead of marking off
the days on the calendar. **BEECH** is also a useful remedy,
sometimes going hand in hand with **IMPATIENS** if you
feel generally irritated by people's presence.

As the long awaited date draws ever nearer, you may also
find yourself feeling anxious or afraid of what it will actually
be like (especially if it is your first pregnancy); a time when
panic may set in, or doubts about whether it will be "alright"
or whether the baby will be normal and healthy. After all,
when one stops to really think about it, that rather large
pregnancy, the bulk of which is solid baby, has to emerge
through what seems to be a very small orifice! It can indeed be

frightening and if you are unprepared, your imagination can begin to run riot and dream up all sorts of horrific scenarios. **ROCK ROSE** is the remedy to help ease terrifying thoughts; **MIMULUS** for less severe, known fears; **WHITE CHESTNUT** if you cannot release your mind from niggling worries; **ASPEN** for apprehension and a sense of uneasiness; **CHERRY PLUM** for the imagination that plays havoc with rational thoughts.

Many women ask whether it is safe to take the Remedies during pregnancy. They are quite harmless and so cannot cause any ill-effects and therefore considered to be entirely safe. They do, however, contain brandy which is included as a preservative, so they should be taken diluted. If you are in any doubt at all, then it would always be sensible to have a word with your midwife who will put your mind at rest.

LABOUR AND CHILDBIRTH

During the course of your pregnancy, it is usual to have had at least one ultrasound scan. This simple and painless technique is a very useful means of determining the baby's gestational age, although a series of scans will provide the most accurate information about its progress and rate of growth. If you have not kept a record of your last period, an expected date of delivery will have been difficult to assess, and in this case, a scan will be a very helpful way of predicting when the baby will be due.

Pregnancy lasts for 38 weeks from conception, but because the age of the pregnancy is calculated from the date of the last menstrual period, it is said to be of 40 weeks duration. If your pregnancy continues beyond 40 weeks, you will be monitored more closely as a safeguard to prevent any complications. There is a lot to be said for leaving nature to its own devices, and not interfering in the course of events – childbirth is a natural process after all, not a medical condition. If labour does not start when it is scheduled to, it may simply be because the time is not right, and the baby will come when it is ready. If this is the case, there is no reason why there should be any intervention if the baby is healthy and the pregnancy is developing normally. However, after term, the placenta gradually begins to degenerate and as this is the baby's life-line, there may be a risk if the pregnancy goes on for too long. There are however, tests which can be carried out to determine the state of health of the placenta. If signs of placental decline are indicated, there are various ways and means of monitoring the baby's continued well-being, but the doctor or midwife may at this stage begin to talk to you about inducing labour artificially, although they will wait as long as possible, whilst it is safe to do so, for it to begin spontaneously.

Most women have their babies in hospital although some are given the opportunity to opt for a home birth if they so wish. Usually, first babies are delivered in hospital to mini-mise any risk to the mother or infant. This is because until a woman has given birth to one full term baby, it will not be absolutely certain that a vaginal delivery will be possible. This may sound a little obscure, but when you consider that the baby's head which (normally) measures 9.5 centimetres in diameter and 13.5 cms in length, has to pass through a pelvic opening of 11 cms × 13 cms, it is quite a tight fit! As the foetus descends during the last weeks of pregnancy and more especially during labour itself, the bones of the skull overlap slightly (they do not fuse together until the child is about 18 months old, and the "soft spot" felt on a baby's head is the space left where the bones meet, allowing them to overlap during birth), the chin tucks up against the chest and the head twists slightly so that the narrowest diameter of the head passes through the pelvis. It is therefore the back of the head (occiput) that emerges first. The mechanics are quite wonderful, but occasionally a problem will arise if, for example, the head is not flexed sufficiently, is facing forwards instead of backwards, if there is a hand or arm tucked up against the head, or if the baby is particularly large, or the pelvis particularly small. Although unusual, all these things will reduce the pelvic space available and there is a risk of the baby becoming "stuck" which would necessitate a forceps delivery or an emergency Caesarean section – not something that can be performed at home – and clearly, it is preferable that a mother in this position should be where all the necessary emergency facilities are readily available – in the next room, not half an hour away!

It should be stressed at this stage that **abnormalities** occuring during pregnancy, labour and childbirth are the **exceptions** – they are **un**usual. It is a normal natural process and nine times out of ten will progress in a normal and natural way, so do not be too alarmed! It is, however, helpful to be aware of what **might** happen and why, so that if it does, you can feel, at least a little, prepared for it.

So . . . assuming all will be well, and that you have been admitted to hospital, either because labour has started spontaneously, or because it is felt appropriate to induce it artificially, what happens next? There is generally a "procedure" which includes an examination to ascertain how far your labour has progressed. If there is time, you will take a bath and change into a gown. You may also have been given something to help you empty your bowels – every millimetre of room within your pelvis is precious! The examination will include a vaginal and abdominal assessment. The vaginal examination is explained below. The abdominal examination is similar to that which you will have experienced at antenatal clinic. The baby's lie can be clarified by feeling the position of the spine, bottom and head (although the latter will not be palpable once it has descended into the pelvis), and its heartbeat heard through a stethoscope, fetoscope (the trumpet-shaped instrument), or via a monitor. At some stage during labour you may be attached to the monitor, perhaps just for a short period so that a record of the baby's heartbeat can be obtained. The monitor also registers the strength and frequency of contractions. These signals are picked up via plates, strapped to your abdomen. It is not painful and nothing to be afraid of, but is somewhat uncomfortable and restraining.

Hospitals are very clinical places and it can all seem rather daunting, especially if you are not used to them, or do not like them. Sometimes just the thought of going to hospital as the due date approaches, can be frightening, creating apprehension and anxiety. If, once admitted, you are faced with monitors and other pieces of unfamiliar equipment, anxiety can easily grow, especially if you were not prepared and did not know what to expect. There are three remedies of particular help on such occasions – **MIMULUS** for fear of known things – hospitals, pain etc., **ASPEN** the unspecific fear of the unknown; apprehension, or dread. The third remedy is **WHITE CHESTNUT** which is for worrying thoughts that go round and round in the mind; whenever you stop what you are doing and allow your mind to **think**, back come the worries . . . White Chestnut is a wonderful remedy for putting the brakes on runaway thoughts and restoring peace of mind.

Some hospitals are able to offer a "family room" which is well worth considering and enquiring about because it makes an ideal compromise between home and hospital – the best of both worlds – providing the comfort and privacy of a room furnished in a homely way, but with all the hosptial back-up just outside the door. These family rooms generally have to be booked in advance because there are usually only one or two, and even then it is largely luck of the draw whether it is occupied already when you need it. It does however, go a long way towards achieving a relaxed and comfortable environment which in itself, will help you to put all those well-practised relaxation techniques into operation!

At the onset of labour, the muscular walls of the uterus begin to contract putting pressure on the baby and forcing its descent. Contractions are generally weak to begin with, becoming stronger as time passes. They also increase in frequency and duration, starting off at about one every twenty minutes and lasting for about 20 seconds, to three or four every ten minutes and lasting for about a minute each time. Each time a contraction occurs, there is a permanent shortening of the muscle fibres, so that the uterus makes itself smaller and smaller. The waves of contractions start at the top where they are strongest, and spread downwards where they are weaker, allowing the lower segment, including the tight rings of muscle around the cervix, to relax. The effect of these persistent waves cause the opening of the cervix (the os) to dilate, opening up the canal through which the baby will be born. When the midwife examines a woman during labour, she will be able to feel the diameter of the os, measuring the opening with her fingers and thus be able to

CERVICAL DILATATION DURING LABOUR

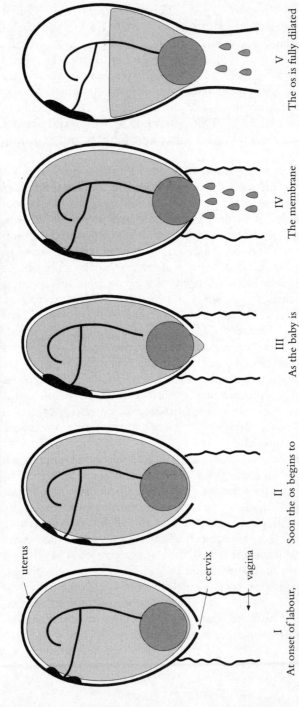

uterus

cervix

vagina

I
At onset of labour, cervical os is still closed

II
Soon the os begins to open causing a release of the plug of mucus which is often blood stained – 'The show'

III
As the baby is pushed down by the contracting uterus, some of the liquor is trapped between the cervix and the baby's head

IV
The membrane ruptures and the pocket of water escapes

V
The os is fully dilated creating an open shaft through which the baby descends

tell how far labour has progressed. It is measured in terms of centimetres, and altogether will expand to 10cm in diameter. The first three centimetres are quite slow as labour is establishing itself, but after that, the os expands rapidly at the rate of approximately 1cm per hour. As the opening reaches full dilatation, the urge to push may be quite overwhelming. Sometimes the midwife will ask you "not to push just yet" – the hardest thing in the world! – but the reason for this is because the cervix has not yet completely effaced, and the tough muscular ring surrounding it is still protruding. There is a risk that this might be damaged if too much pressure is put on it too soon. As the cervix opens, the plug of mucus that has been lodged within it is expelled, and this is sometimes stained with blood. Quite often, this is the first sign that labour has begun, or it may be a sudden feeling of wetness which indicates that the membrane encapsulating the baby in the womb has ruptured, allowing some of the liquor to escape. It is a common worry with mothers who experience this at an early stage, that **all** the liquor has escaped and that the baby is no longer floating in its protective waters. However, this is not the case. The wetness felt is only a small amount of water which has become trapped in front of the baby's head (see diagram). There is no way of knowing which sign – contraction, show of mucus or flow of water – will come first. Every woman and every pregnancy is different.

The period from the onset of labour – that is the onset of regular contractions – to the point when the cervical os is fully dilated, is called the **FIRST STAGE** of labour. For a woman who is experiencing childbirth for the first time, this will last, on average, between 6 and 12 hours. For women who have had a previous child, the first stage is much quicker and will be expected to last only about 4–8 hours. There are, however, always exceptions to the rule. I remember, as a student midwife, one particular lady who was having her fifth baby. As soon as her labour started, she came straight to the hospital, and it was just as well she did because the baby was born before she had a chance to undress! It was my job to meet her when she first arrived, and on our way up to the ward, my heart was pounding as I pictured the awful scenario of me conducting my first delivery in the lift! You can imagine how I felt when she said she wanted to push – and with no Rescue Remedy on me either!

The **SECOND STAGE** of labour begins when the cervix is fully dilated and ends when the baby has been born. This stage takes approximately 30 minutes to an hour in a woman having her first baby, and once again, it is quicker for women who have previously had a child, taking only 5–30 minutes. The uterine contractions are at their strongest at this stage and the baby is pushed down through the open passage which has been formed, linking the uterine cavity with the outside world.

The **THIRD STAGE** of labour begins with the birth of the baby and ends with the safe delivery of the placenta. This only takes between 3 and 10 minutes and usually goes by with minimal awareness – the proud mother being too elated (and exhausted!) to take any notice.

It is probably during the first stage of labour that the Remedies are most needed – **RESCUE REMEDY** in particular. There is no denying that labour is painful. As the contractions increase in strength, so the pain becomes stronger. You will have been given the opportunity to practise breathing techniques during mothercraft/parentcraft or ante-natal classes, and these exercises are designed to help you to remain in control; to help encourage a "mind over matter" approach. It does, however, take quite a lot of self-control to maintain a calm breathing pattern throughout, and it can be all too easy to give in to the almighty surge of constriction and pain and go to pieces as a result. This is when it really becomes an ordeal and the desperation of not knowing, or believing when or if it will ever end can be agonizing, and feelings of anger, resentment or even hatred towards the midwife and unborn infant – the cause of pain – may begin to creep into the mind. Ironically, this stress, tension, panic and loss of control all have a hindering effect on the progress of labour, as mental tension quickly results in physical tension. As we have seen, during a contraction, the lower segment of the uterus including the cervix, becomes softer and more relaxed. If muscle fibres become tense and rigid as a result of becoming worked up emotionally, the softening and dilatation of the cervical os will be countered by the tension which is being created in the muscles.

Clearly, the thing to do is to break into that cycle of events. Pain relief itself will ease the physical tension which will in turn relieve some of the emotional strain, and there is nothing to feel guilty about or any reason to consider yourself weak in any way should you feel you need some form of pain relief. Each one of us has our individual pain threshold, and so some women are therefore able to tolerate less pain than others. This is not a sign of weakness or strength, simply a difference in genetic make-up – just as some people have a larger appetite than others. However, the mental outlook is a most important factor, and helping the mind remain calm and in control will help to prevent the series of events that can quickly become counter-productive once heightened anxiety and surmounting fear are allowed to take the upper hand. **RESCUE REMEDY** is the ideal remedy during this time. Four drops added to a glass of water which can be sipped at intervals every so often during the first stage of labour will help to ease the panic or shock, and is altogether calming. Labour will not be pain free, but as the remedy helps you to remain mentally in control, this will in turn help it to progress unhindered by overpowering emotional strain.

RESCUE REMEDY can be continued after the baby has been born, if necessary, and it will help your system in its recovery. **WALNUT** is also a helpful remedy to include at this stage because this is the remedy for periods of change, and childbirth is one of the most dramatic changes your body will experience. For your newborn child, it is also a period of great adjustment and so if you are breast feeding, your baby will gain the benefit of the remedy too.

Once you have your baby safely in your arms, the memory of those hours in labour, all the pain and the anguish, soon drift into the back of the mind, replaced by the surge of a new emotion – the wonder and pure joy of motherhood. Indeed it is a wonderful moment, and I can recall vividly the first baby I ever saw delivered. It was the most marvellous and beautiful thing I had ever seen, and very humbling too, as you realise with the evidence there before your eyes, the incredible enormity and completeness of nature. So complex, yet awesome in its simplicity.

> "He on whom
> God's light
> does fall
> sees
> the great things
> in the small."

> Piet Hein 1959

POST-NATALLY

So far, with the exception of a few anomalies, we have considered a normal healthy pregnancy, ending in the birth of a normal healthy baby which is both wanted and welcomed. Ideally this is how it should be, and in most instances this is indeed how it is, but even in such happy circumstances, once the euphoria of the first few days has subsided, and consistent with a rapid decline in the levels of hormones progesterone and oestrogen in your system, elation can quickly become deflation, resulting in the notorious "baby blues". This depression of spirits is common and quite normal, but nonetheless disturbing. It varies from one woman to another as to how severe this depression might be and how long it will last. It is usually something that lifts after a few days and indeed some women do not suffer with it at all, but it can go on much longer and very occasionally might develop into what is termed "post-natal psychosis", but let us not get too concerned with terms. What is important is how to cope with it if it comes, and what you can do to help yourself. The Bach Remedies, although very gentle, can certainly be of great help and if taken straight away, before the depression has had a chance to really dig its heels in, so much the better.

We all have our own individual personalities and characters, and so it follows that we should treat ourselves in an individual way, choosing remedies according to **WHO** we are, **HOW** we are and **WHY** we feel the way we do.

Depression itself is a blanket term – it is not specific and does not actually **describe** the feeling on a personal level. It can mean different things to different people – some may consider being in a bad mood, irritable or fed up as being depressed; others may consider it to be self-pity; for others nothing less than suicidal despair would be classed as "depression". Depression itself, means a lowering of the spirits – feeling down; unhappy. There can, however, be any number of causes – failing an interview or examination, receiving some bad news, ending a relationship, having your wallet stolen – there may not even **BE** a reason; it may descend out of the blue for no reason whatsoever, yet be equally miserable, if not more so. There may be an actual reason for post-natal depression that is superimposed upon the hormonal trough – something connected with the birth of the child, or something external, totally unconnected. The classic post-natal depression however, seems to descend for no apparent reason, sometimes falling on those who are overjoyed with their baby, have a loving husband and a secure home, and yet a cloud of gloom overshadows it all. For these women it can be particularly difficult to fathom because there is nothing to account for it, no cause to attach to it, and thus all the harder to accept. The remedy for this kind of depression is **MUSTARD** and it gently helps to remove the heavy cloud, allowing happiness to return. If, however, the reason for the depression is known – for example you have had stitches and find them uncomfortable, or your baby has to spend a little time in the special care baby unit; because you have to stay in hospital longer than you wanted to, or because your husband/partner tells you that the car has broken down beyond repair – when you feel disappointed or disheartened, then **GENTIAN** is the remedy you need to help you feel more encouraged and positive. If, however, the reason for the depression is something of greater depth; something serious that fills you with despair, then **SWEET CHESTNUT** is the remedy to help you. If the depression frightens you as though you might be losing control of your mind, or it makes you feel the urge to do something to harm yourself or your baby, then **CHERRY PLUM** is the remedy to help relieve such intense and frightening feelings. For guilt having felt that way, **PINE** is the remedy to help you cope with this back-lash. **CLEMATIS** would be indicated if you feel that you are not "grounded", feel in a dream world as though what is going on around you is not really happening, making you feel detached from reality. **CLEMATIS** is also indicated if your imagination runs away with you and makes you drift into a world of fantasy. It will bring you back to the here and now, so that those precious moments with your newborn baby do not drift by unnoticed.

Concern for your baby is natural, but if you feel that you are **over**-anxious and fearful about your baby's well-being, then **RED CHESTNUT** will help to allay those fears and put them into true perspective. **STAR OF BETHLEHEM** is another helpful remedy to consider. It is the remedy for shock and will help you to recover, especially if the delivery has been traumatic. For your baby too, this remedy will help to ease the shock of a difficult birth, and in combination with **WALNUT**, will make the transition into our world that much easier.

If you have had stitches, it is important to keep the area clean and dry to prevent infection. You may like to add a few drops of **RESCUE REMEDY** and **CRAB APPLE** to the water when you bathe or wash. Rescue Remedy will help to ease the trauma and the Crab Apple will act as a cleanser, thus promoting your own natural healing. The application of **RESCUE REMEDY CREAM** would also be very soothing.

The most natural way for a mother to feed her baby is at the breast. Breast milk contains all the necessary nutrients in exactly the right proportions for the baby's requirements during its first weeks of life. Not every woman finds breast feeding comfortable and not every woman produces sufficient milk to satisfy her baby. However, if you can, it will not only provide your infant with the food it is intended to have, it will also give you the satisfaction of watching your baby grow on the strength of the nourishment you have provided. The closeness and that special relationsip you share, will also cement the bond between you. If you cannot breast feed for one reason or another, however, you should not feel guilty or reproach yourself. Not every woman finds it a pleasurable experience, and some find the sensation intolerable. If this is the case, I do not believe there is any benefit to be gained by forcing the issue as it merely makes it worse. If you are stressed or under pressure, then your baby will sense your agitation and will also be fretful. Feeding time then becomes an anxious ordeal instead of a relaxed and enjoyable occasion. If you should feel guilty (although you really shouldn't), **PINE** is the remedy to help you remove the blame you have attached to yourself.

During the first two or three days, only a small quantity of milky substance is produced and some women worry that they are not producing sufficient milk. However, this is quite normal. The first substance produced from the breast is called "colostrum" and although it is not produced in large quantities, it is highly nutritious and also contains antibodies which will help to protect your baby from infection. The milk "comes in" on about the third day, and your breasts may feel very tender due to the expanding milk cells and venous congestion. However, once feeding and the flow of milk is established, the breasts will feel more comfortable.

If your nipples should become sore, this may be because the baby is not attaching its mouth to your breast properly, and therefore clasping the actual nipple rather than the areola, or it may simply be due to over-zealous suckling! **RESCUE REMEDY CREAM** because it is so soothing and healing, can be extremely helpful for sore nipples. Apply it as often as necessary, but especially after feeds and at the end of the day. Before a feed, simply clean your breasts in the usual way, and this will remove the residue of the cream.

CHAPTER FIVE

When Pregnancy Does Not Go According To Plan

In this chapter we are going to consider some other aspects of pregnancy and childbirth that do not have such happy endings, or beginnings, and the emotional turbulence and implications surrounding them.

I. AN UNWANTED PREGNANCY

We discussed in Chapter Two how, when we first commence a serious relationship, the biggest "dread" of all is becoming pregnant. This feeling, however, is not confined solely to youth; it may be something that extends well into a woman's thirties and forties. Not every woman wants to have children, but there are many other reasons too that may be the basis of anxiety. There may be fear associated with the physical changes, discomfort or pain, or perhaps pregnancy is considered a threat to a career, freedom or lifestyle, or perhaps it would cause financial strain. For whatever reason, there is always a niggling worry that the chosen contraceptive might fail, unless, of course, you or your partner has been sterilized, and so it is difficult to feel completely relaxed.

If, therefore, pregnancy should occur when you really do

not want to be pregnant, then the news may be devastating and generate all kinds of emotions. The first of these will, more than likely, be shock, horror or disbelief. **STAR OF BETHLEHEM** is the remedy to help ease the initial trauma. It may be followed by feelings of anger, mixed with worry and anxiety about what to do next, and then as the full impact is absorbed, the reality of the situation becomes evident and as it does, the full implications of what it all actually means. Depending on the situation, the stability of the relationship and the partner's feelings, the diagnosis will present a more difficult problem for some than for others. Some couples may adjust and be able to come to terms with the idea; perhaps the maternal surge of emotions will alter the outlook on life, whilst for others it will not. Some couples may disagree with one another – one partner surprised but pleased and prepared to adjust, the other adamant that a baby would be an intrusion on their life and looked upon as the beginning of the end. This conflict, over such an important issue, can in itself disturb even the soundest relationships and may be disastrous for those which are less stable. Although there may be some explosive feelings vented in the beginning, it is really something which should be discussed together; rationally and seriously. It involves a new life; a life that has already begun, but also affects your own life, and so whatever you decide to do, it should be thought about carefully before taking one route or another. Looking at the situation like this in an objective way, it is clearly a delicate dilemma and it goes without saying that whatever decision is made, it should not be taken unless you are sure that that is what you really want to do. However, looking at a hypothetical situation is one thing; being personally involved in it is quite another, and it is by no means unusual to find logical thought and clarity of mind deserting you, and no matter how hard you try, all that fills your head are feelings of panic, despair, wild imaginings and confusion. It is then difficult to see the way forward clearly enough to make a decision at all, let alone the right one.

In reality there are two avenues to take – two choices. One is to accept the pregnancy and readjust your plans and your life to include a (or another) baby. The alternative is to have the pregnancy terminated. This may sound rather a cold harsh choice, perhaps too black and white, and indeed it may not seem at all as clear cut as that. All sorts of grey areas may surround the decision you are trying to make, but the bottom line remains the same, and ultimately the choice between these two avenues is what you will have to make. It is a big decision and certainly not the easiest. Ironically, it is one which really needs a lot of thought, and yet because you do not have time on your side, it is one which has to be made quickly, often before there is time to think about it properly: if a pregnancy is going to be terminated, this will need to be done early, ideally within the first twelve weeks. If you are a person who has not been in the habit of keeping a record of period dates, then you may not realise you are pregnant until the pregnancy has developed to several weeks, maybe longer, and so not only do you have to make an almighty decision about what to do about it, you have to contend with doing so whilst still feeling shocked or stunned by the knowledge of the result you have just received.

If you do not want to be pregnant; if you do not want a baby, then the logical thing to do in the circumstances may be to opt for a termination of pregnancy. However, bringing it to an end may be something that is desired, but not considered a realistic option because of certain beliefs or moral values that you hold. Every woman, every couple, have their own ideas and opinions about when life really begins, and so for some, abortion may be considered to be distasteful, wrong, wicked; whereas for others, a pregnancy consisting of only a ball of cells or early embryo might not be thought of as "alive" in the true sense of the word – certainly it would be unable to support its own life at that stage – and for those who feel this way, the question marks surrounding whether it is right or wrong to terminate a pregnancy may not exist.

If you have strong opinions either way, then the decision will not be so difficult. If, however, you find yourself torn between what you think you ought to do and what you feel you really **want** to do, then the dilemma can be bitterly traumatic. If you should feel that the common sense approach is to consider your future, your career, your independence and so on, yet have doubts in your mind, then making up your mind to bring the pregnancy to an end will need to be supported by a lot of self-reassurance, counter-arguments, advantages over disadvantages and so on in order to convince yourself that this is what you really **want** to do; that without a shadow of doubt it is for the best. The emotional whirlpool can be extremely strong and all too easy to be engulfed by. If your heart is telling you "no", then to go ahead with an abortion will be very difficult to come to terms with later, even when it is all over. Nothing will really be the same again – time cannot be turned back, and to kid yourself that it can, may be the most upsetting and uncomfortable mistake you could make. Feelings of guilt and grief can, for some women, be overwhelming, and even if a very firm decision has been made, it may still arouse emotions that you least expect. Sometimes these feelings can linger on for years and may never be really overcome – something that haunts you, always there at the back of your mind. There are, nevertheless, circumstances that force this difficult choice upon a woman; circumstances that would make life for everyone concerned, including the new baby, hazardous or at the very least, worrying and unhappy. You may therefore have to make the decision to end the pregnancy, not because you want to, but because you know it would not be fair on either of you to continue with it. Or perhaps the decision has been reached because your own health is threatened, or perhaps the baby would be born damaged in some way. In circumstances like this, the decision to have an abortion can be extremely disconcerting, and desperately unhappy and we will be discussing this in a little more detail later in this chapter.

However, whatever the reasons, the emotions surrounding it may be the same and because they are so powerful, they have the potential to linger for a long time. There are, however, many remedies that can be suggested, and by taking the right one at the right time, much of the emotional anguish that may otherwise follow, can be avoided and replaced by more positive thoughts about the future.

PINE is the remedy for feelings of guilt; **STAR OF BETHLEHEM** for shock and grief, a feeling that can be quite overwhelming and a surprise to encounter if unprepared; **CRAB APPLE** for self-hatred, self-disgust, feeling unclean, contaminated or interfered with. These are remedies that would be appropriate, where necessary, afterwards, but let us turn our attention once more to the weeks beforehand, the period during which you are trying to reach a clear decision. This is the time when the Remedies can be of the greatest relief, because they have the chance to act in a preventative manner, allowing you to deal with the feelings, and thus take the first step towards making your choice with confidence and peace of mind. This will then negate all the turbulence that may otherwise follow.

Remedies to consider are those which deal not only with the moods and emotions that are experienced, but also for your basic temperament because it is undoubtedly the sort of person you are – your underlying nature – that gives rise to the dilemma in the first place. Let us consider some examples.

CRAB APPLE for the feeling that makes you uncomfortable, as though you have something growing inside you that you do not like; as though you are playing host to a parasite.

STAR OF BETHLEHEM for shock – the sudden unexpected realisation; feeling stunned or numb.

SCLERANTHUS if you are finding it hard to come to a decision – first considering one option and then another, unable to choose between the two. Scleranthus is the remedy to ease this mental ping-pong and allow your mind to settle once and for all on one side of the fence or the other.

CERATO if you find yourself having made a decision, perhaps even a sub-conscious one, but then distrusting it; having insufficient belief in yourself to really trust and have faith in your decision. Thus you find that you need to ask someone else what they think you should do; looking and hoping for someone or something who will make up your mind for you. You may find yourself, in this state of mind, taking the advice of others or taking notice of people's opinions that go against your own, and yet find yourself trusting them more than you trust your own intuition. This sort of self-doubt needs Cerato and the remedy will help you to be more certain about yourself and to know and understand your own mind.

WALNUT if you are normally quite set upon your own direction; someone who has a clear idea about what you want, where you are going and what to do, but at times such as this, find yourself being influenced by the opinions of others. Not that you have sought them, as in Cerato above, but have had them thrust upon you nevertheless. Having received them, you feel unable to shake them off, as though they have diverted you from your usual clarity and chosen route. Walnut is the remedy to help you to withstand such powerful outside influences and keep yourself apart from them. It is also a very helpful remedy for periods of change and adjustment, so if you are finding it hard to come to terms with the news, or find it difficult to adjust to the step you have decided to take, Walnut will help you to feel more settled.

CENTAURY – this remedy will help those who are easily dominated by the strong will of others; for those who succumb to more forceful characters and who in a situation like this may find that their decision is made for them – perhaps by a parent or partner with a stronger personality. Centaury is the remedy to provide gentle people such as this with more strength to stand up for themselves and to do what **they** want to do, rather than what someone else thinks would be good for them.

MIMULUS – This remedy is for fear of known things, for nervousness, or shyness. It is helpful for people of this nature but also helpful for anyone who suffers with fear – fear of making a mistake, fear of not being able to cope, or feeling afraid to confide in someone in case the reaction is unpleasant. This remedy will provide a gentle courage to overcome these anxieties, and help the sufferer put them into perspective and face them with a greater sense of security and assurance.

ASPEN – this remedy is also for fear, but instead of being of known origin, the Aspen fear is one of apprehension – vague unknown fears, not clearly defined, that can be very disturbing and worsened simply because it is impossible to identify their cause.

ELM if you are a person who is normally capable and confident who copes well with responsibility, but faced with the awesome responsibility of a new life growing inside you, and the decision about its future, you feel overwhelmed with it all, begin to doubt your ability to cope and start to lose faith in yourself. Elm will help to restore your confidence and capabilities and help you feel more in control of the situation.

GENTIAN for disappointment and a depressed feeling due to the situation or circumstances surrounding it. This remedy gives encouragement and promotes a more positive outlook on life.

Just by taking the right remedy or mixture of remedies to help you see your way forward more clearly, you may realise that having a baby, although it may not be convenient at the present time, only takes adjustment. The prospect of being pregnant, once you become used to the idea, can then become a joyful one, something to look upon as a blessing; something to enrich your life. Conversely, you may come to the conclusion that a baby is definitely not what you want and feel equally confident and self-assured. Whatever decision you make, being able to think about it more clearly will enable you to make the right decision for **YOU** – whatever that may be – and have no regrets, no doubts, and thus avoid the inevitable heartache that making the wrong choice would bring.

II. LOSING A PREGNANCY; LOSING A BABY

The loss of a pregnancy through miscarriage or the loss of a baby through a very premature labour can be extremely difficult to live with or even comprehend. A dearly wanted baby, especially if the couple have been trying to conceive for some time, ending in miscarriage can be devastating, and the heartache tremendous. Even if the pregnancy ends very early on before the foetus has developed any shape or detail, the traumas of its loss may be equally as great as that taking place in later pregnancy. Losing a baby after about twenty weeks is nevertheless, in most instances, a much greater shock. By this time, a woman has had a chance to feel her baby moving, kicking, growing; she has experienced her own body changes both emotionally and physically. The baby is part of her, dependent on her, and even before she sees it, a strong bond between mother and baby is developing. Plans are made for the baby's arrival – clothes will have been given or bought or knitted, a cradle, carry-cot or pram will have been considered if not actually obtained, and thoughts about where the baby will sleep, equipment for feeding and travelling will all have entered the mind. For all these plans to suddenly be brought to an end, and for the insurmountable pain of losing the baby – losing the feeling inside, the physical symptoms, the pregnant bulge, the contentment, the glow – all to vanish in a moment is bewildering. Like a bubble bursting, or the bottom falling out of a wonderful and happy world, and with only confusion and anguish to replace it.

Premature Labour
By about 20 weeks of pregnancy, the foetus looks unmistakably like a baby – it is virtually completely formed. At 28 weeks the baby is considered to be viable, that is, it has the potential to survive unaided outside the mother's body. This, however, does not mean that a baby born before this time cannot live. Babies born before 28 weeks often do survive but they do need special care – incubation, special feeding techniques and special breathing apparatus and monitoring to help them during these early weeks.

Babies born at any time before about 37 weeks are likely to need some special attention, and even full term babies may require some time in the Special Care Baby Unit if they have had a difficult birth.

Let us consider some Remedies that may be helpful:
STAR OF BETHLEHEM to ease the trauma; **MIMULUS**

for fear and nervousness – this may be particularly helpful for you if your baby is being cared for in an incubator because it is only natural to feel afraid when surrounded by high-tech equipment, and sterile techniques, and it can be quite unnerving to hold a baby so small. That first time is always an anxious moment, afraid of hurting its delicate little body. It is, however, a matter of becoming used to handling your tiny baby, and it is important that you do because it will help overcome your fear and cement the bond between you. If you find yourself becoming over-anxious; your fears and worries out of proportion, then the remedy you need is **RED CHESTNUT**. This will help the exaggerated concerns you have for your baby's safety become contained and rational. If you should find it hard to escape from disturbing and worrying thoughts, then **WHITE CHESTNUT** will make an excellent complement to the other remedies you may need as it helps to re-establish peace of mind.

Sometimes the equipment surrounding a young pre-term baby can be off-putting. We have discussed the way it can instil fear, especially if it has not been explained thoroughly enough to you, as it will then always be shrouded in mystery and inevitably create further anxiety. We have also discussed how important it is to maintain close contact with your baby during this time so as to develop and reinforce your natural bond. There is, however, another angle to a premature infant's technological and clinical environment, and that is alienation. It is, naturally, more difficult to really get to know your baby because it is not with you constantly, to tend to, to pick up and comfort when it cries, or even to feed in the normal way. All these things, in addition to the awe-inspiring monitors, may make you feel that the child you see does not really belong to you; you may feel emotionless, totally detached from it. If you should feel like this, there are a number of remedies that can be helpful, depending on exactly how it affects you. **WILD ROSE** will help the resignation and emotional flatness; **SWEET CHESTNUT** if you feel an inner overwhelming despair; **GORSE** if you have given up hope and feel very pessimistic about the future; **WILLOW** if you feel resentful towards life, or towards your child for having been so inconsiderate by demanding to be born so soon. Alternatively you may feel tremendous guilt and blame yourself for the prematurity of your infant, believing that you must have done something to have caused it, that you could have prevented it. If you feel like this, then **PINE** is the remedy you need to help you overcome these feelings of self-reproach, and to appreciate that life has a habit of being so unpredictable that it is not in our hands to determine what will happen. If you feel a gulf between you; a barrier you cannot penetrate – if you feel detached or unmoved, then **WATER VIOLET** would be helpful; or **WILD ROSE** as mentioned above, if you feel neither happy nor sad, but apathetically accepting whatever lies in store. This remedy may also be helpful if you should feel that you are just "going through the motions" unable to express or even feel any emotion.

CLEMATIS would also be helpful and more appropriate if you feel as though you are living in a dream, as though what is going on around you is not really happening; perhaps you find your thoughts drifting into some fantasy imagining some happier circumstance; feeling totally disinterested in the reality of the moment. There is also, of course, the element of shock which may give rise to similar feelings, and in this case **STAR OF BETHLEHEM** should be added. Both Clematis and Star of Bethlehem are ingredients of the **RESCUE REMEDY**, and so this would be particularly helpful initially.

Miscarriage

Theoretically, any pregnancy that ends before it has reached 28 weeks, and the baby has not been born alive, is termed a miscarriage. We have already discussed how agonizing later miscarriages can be, but early miscarriages can be equally traumatic.

However, because they occur before the baby has had a chance to really develop and been felt to move, it is generally a little easier to cope with. We usually consider miscarriage as something that occurs **after** pregnancy has been confirmed, marked by severe lower abdominal pain and heavy bleeding, rather like an extremely uncomfortable period. However, miscarriages can occur before a woman even knows she is pregnant and would not consider that she had experienced anything other than normal menstrual bleeding. A large number of pregnancies are thought to end this way – it would simply be a conceived pregnancy that has either not implanted into the body of the uterus, or one that has divided abnormally after fertilization. The egg cell is therefore expelled from the uterus in the normal way, followed by a decline in the hormone progesterone and shedding of the endometrium. This would happen either at the expected time of the period, or perhaps a few days later, and is nature's way of ensuring that only healthy, viable embryos survive and mature. We usually consider miscarriage, however, as the loss of a pregnancy after it has been established for a few weeks. The most common time for miscarriages to occur is at the time when the normal menstrual period would otherwise be due – i.e. at 4, 8 and 12 weeks. These first three months are the most precarious, and once past the 12 week mark, the pregnancy is considered to be more stable. Some women experience habitual miscarriages (the term used for those who have had at least 3), and so a closer eye will be kept on subsequent pregnancies, and more than average rest recommended. Slight bleeding is not uncommon, especially at the normal period milestones, but this should be painless and very light, and only last for a few hours or a couple of days at the most. Some women have been reported to experience this kind of bleeding for virtually the duration of their pregnancy and if menstruation is light ordinarily, this bleeding may be mistaken for a normal period, and pregnancy not suspected or diagnosed until it has become more obvious. However, although slight bleeding is not uncommon, it is not exactly "normal" and so if it should occur, the woman should rest in bed until it stops, and then take things very gently. Always avoid lifting heavy objects – heavy bags of shopping for example, or even the vacuum cleaner – during pregnancy, but more particularly if you have bled or have had a previous miscarriage. There is no need to become an invalid or treat yourself like a fragile ornament, but all bleeding in early pregnancy should be considered a "threatened miscarriage" and precautionary measures to preserve it taken accordingly.

The words "miscarriage" and "abortion" mean the same thing, although miscarriage is generally used for a pregnancy that ends spontaneously, whilst abortion is generally reserved for pregnancies that are terminated therapeutically. A spontaneous abortion can either be threatened or inevitable, and if inevitable, may be either complete or incomplete. An incomplete abortion or miscarriage means that some contents of conception remain in the uterus. This will cause prolonged bleeding which may be severe and may cause infection, resulting in a variety of complications possibly hindering future pregnancy attempts. This is why it is important, if you do miscarry, to always seek medical attention. This way, you can be thoroughly examined to ensure that nothing has been left behind. If there has, or some products of conception are suspected to have been retained, then a small operation may be performed to remove the last fragments of tissue and thus avoid complications.

Miscarriages can occur for several different reasons. Habitual abortions are most often due to either an incompetent cervix – i.e. the muscular bands that keep it tightly closed are not as strong as they should be, perhaps weakened by previous gynaecological surgery or during previous childbirth – or due to abnormalities of the uterus itself, making it difficult for the fertilized ovum to embed itself or, if it does, for the pregnancy to grow normally. Other causes include high fever, renal disease, diabetes, severe anaemia, syphilis, genetic and other abnormalities of the foetus, or severe emotional shock. Perhaps it is nature's way of dealing with one thing at a time and ensuring the well-being of the mother before allowing a pregnancy to continue.

Ectopic pregnancies, those which occur outside the uterine cavity, usually embedding in the wall of the Fallopian tube rather than in the wall of the uterus, should be diagnosed as early as possible because complications of haemorrhage and shock can be serious. Ectopic pregnancies however, do not usually go by unnoticed because the symptoms are, in themselves, quite severe – fainting attacks, pain and watery bleeding which might be superimposed upon a normal period.

Whatever the causes or physical symptoms, the primary emotional consideration, is shock. **STAR OF BETH-LEHEM** therefore is the remedy indicated, although **RESCUE REMEDY** is usually more readily to hand and as it contains not only Star of Bethlehem, but **ROCK ROSE** for terror and panic, and **CHERRY PLUM** for loss of emotional control, it may be an even better choice than Star of Bethlehem alone, an invaluable remedy to have on stand by for emergencies.

The Stillborn Baby

Of all the circumstances surrounding losing a baby, losing it in childbirth is the most devastating and something dreaded by most prospective mothers. The loss of a baby, often a full term baby, so suddenly, is bound to cause severe emotional shock, followed by grief and a deep sadness. Understandably post-natal depression can, in such circumstances, be very deep. Counselling is very important, not only for the mother but for the couple as a unit to help them to cope with their loss, generating all the feelings associated with losing someone dear, except that in the case of a stillborn baby, the chance to know it, experience its responses, feed it, change its nappy or look into its eyes, have been denied – all the things that have been looked forward to so much. Grief may be even greater, because there is no clear identity or living memory on which to reflect and deposit one's sorrow. It is therefore important for both the mother and the father to have the opportunity to hold their baby, to cherish it and thus be allowed to grieve naturally for their lost child. Hopefully, a mother who has lost her baby will be able to go home early. It can otherwise be most distressing for her to remain in hospital on a post-natal ward with all the other mothers and their newborn healthy infants. In some cases it may be therapeutic, but for most, it will simply add to the heartache and just serve to reinforce the emptiness. Going home without your baby may be even harder – there will be neighbours, friends and family to face and explain to, people's sympathies and awkwardness to cope with, an empty house, an empty cradle, a drawer of baby clothes lying dormant and useless, and most of all, two people with heavy hearts and empty arms.

To experience something so tragic and to be confronted so closely with life and death, makes one realise just how fragile life can be, and how we can never take it for granted. Fate can seem exceedingly cruel at times, and although one may believe that destiny – life's great plan – has placed such tragedy in our path for a reason, accepting it and living with it as such is much harder work, for despite everything, we only have our human abilities to cope with the reality of the pain and heartache.

Support for one another at a time like this is crucial and the essence of surviving the coming weeks or months. For those coping alone, having someone to turn to is therefore even more important. A friend or close relative would be a great comfort, but unfortunately sometimes there is really no-one to confide in, and although the prospect of seeing a counsellor may seem cold, like meeting a stranger, it is an important step, because while at the end of the day the problem is yours alone, sharing your feelings with someone else goes a long way towards easing the burden from your own mind. It helps to clear the head, leaving room for more encouraging and optimistic thoughts of now and of the future.

Thankfully, the Remedies are there to help ease the turbulent emotions that lurk within, and allow peace to return to the mind and the heart. I am sure Dr. Bach's name has been blessed many, many times for providing such a gentle means of coping with life's traumas, and for showing us the way to learn from them in the unpredictable journey we take through life.

Remedies for bereavement will differ from one person to the next because we all cope with grief in our own personal ways. Nevertheless, the following describes those that are most commonly indicated:

STAR OF BETHLEHEM for the shock, and for the grieving and emptiness – emotions of the heart.

SWEET CHESTNUT – for the despair, heartache and deep depression as though life no longer has anything to offer; feeling ensnared in unhappiness and unable to see any way out that will bring relief.

WALNUT to help ease the difficult readjustment to life.

CRAB APPLE – for a sense of revulsion or an overwhelming desire to rid the body of some presence or influence. This may occur if the baby has died during pregnancy but remains in utero. This sensation can be particularly disturbing.

CHERRY PLUM for irrational thoughts, the mind out of control, or for the feeling of panic as though one might go insane if the nightmare is not brought to an end. It is also the remedy indicated where wild thoughts of suicide enter the mind.

PINE for feelings of guilt and remorse, blaming yourself for the tragedy, and believing that you must have done something terribly wrong.

CLEMATIS for a stunned, distant state of mind as though it is all a dream, happening yet not happening; feeling dazed and numb.

HONEYSUCKLE for the absorption in what has gone, reliving events, lingering memories of how happy it could have been; dwelling on the past and unable to move forward or think about what tomorrow might bring.

WILLOW – for the resentment and bitterness towards life for handing out such harsh treatment; and for any consequential introspective self-pity, especially as you see other mothers with their babies, pushing prams or push-chairs, oblivious of your personal tragedy and seemingly unappreciative of how lucky they are.

HEATHER – for the desire to talk about the experience over and over again, when it dominates the conversation, and even when alone, the thoughts are filled with nothing else.

HOLLY for the angry desire for revenge; despising life and for feelings of hatred or jealousy towards other women who have children. Anger plays a big part in the grieving process and so this remedy, and/or Willow for these feelings are important, although a big soft cushion to "punch the hell out of" can also be very therapeutic!

III. JENNIFER'S STORY

Jennifer consulted us initially because she was worried about her ability to conceive a child and felt that her negative emotions were causing some sort of block. She was a "futuristic" type of person – always needing something to look forward to; always planning ahead, imagining and fantasizing. She could become wrapped up in her own thoughts and frequently allowed her mind to drift. She was a Clematis "type". We treated her with this remedy together with others to help her emotional feelings at that time. She soon regained a positive outlook and continued for the rest of the year to try for a baby, and although her attempts never came to fruition, did not give up and remained hopeful throughout. We did not hear from her for some time after that, but later we learned that she had, in the end, sought medical help which had involved a series of investigations both for herself and her husband, and then commenced treatment to induce ovulation – tablets and injections in increasing doses, and then a combination of the two. Two years later she wrote to us again explaining what had happened since she was last in touch. This is her story.

"Dear Friends,

You might remember me. I have benefited very much from the advice you have given in the past and I thought you might be interested to hear how my life has progressed. I have, as you may recall, been desperately trying to conceive a baby for three years, and have lived in hope month after month only to have those hopes dashed every time. I thought I had reached the stage when I felt I had borne enough anguish and because I had lived with my obsession for such a long time, I actually began to find some sort of solace in coming to terms with childlessness. I started to tell myself, or rather, make myself believe, that perhaps not having children wasn't such a bad thing. Perhaps it even had its benefits – freedom, a life for *us*; we could go anywhere, do anything, get up late if we wanted to, watch a film uninterrupted. . . . I even wondered whether I was destined for motherhood anyway . . .

But then it happened! Just before Christmas my period started as usual, which was naturally upsetting and had me in floods of tears as usual. However, on that occasion it seemd particularly light, only lasting a couple of days. I didn't give this much thought at the time, but then as the days went by, I noticed that instead of the pre-menstrual breast tenderness disappearing with the onset of my period, it continued and seemed to increase. I then began to wonder if I might possibly be pregnant, although I hardly dared tempt fate by allowing my imagination to have too much freedom! I'm afraid I couldn't even summon up the courage to do a pregnancy test, despite the fact that I had had a pack of "Clearblue" for some time in the bathroom cabinet, just waiting for this moment! I simply couldn't bear the disappointment of a negative result and so I therefore decided to hang on to the dream for as long as possible. I did, however, pluck up enough courage to check my temperature. I had been taking it each morning because this was part of my infertility treatment regime, but when my period began I did not bother and had not done so since. I knew that if I was pregnant it would still be raised. So, the next morning, taking a deep breath, I placed the thermometer in my mouth and kept my fingers crossed while my heart thumped rapidly in my chest for the duration of the next few minutes. To my relief and astonishment it was still elevated, and that meant that perhaps I really was . . . I hardly dared to allow my hopes to get too high. I had been through all that before. I decided to ring my gynaecologist – I had to know one way or the other, and as we were going away for Christmas I really couldn't wait any longer. I took a sample of urine with me so that he could perform the pregnancy test I hadn't the courage to do myself. As I waited in his office for the result, I remember thinking "this is worse than taking my driving test"! Those three minutes were among the most agonizingly anxious in my life! What a relief when he eventually came back in, a broad smile on his face, confirming that it was a positive result. I was pregnant! I could hardly believe it. Without a doubt, that was the best Christmas present I could possibly wish to have.

We spent New Year away with some friends. Although a most enjoyable and restful week, I nevertheless felt a little unsafe being so far away from home. When I had a small amount of spotting, which naturally worried and frightened me, I was eager to get home again and anxious for reassurance that all was well. As this was impractical I went straight to bed and hardly dared walk more than a few yards for the rest of the holiday! It was a great shame as I missed out on excursions and thus had little opportunity to appreciate the wonderful countryside and scenic surroundings. Nevertheless, I would have sacrificed a great deal more to ensure a healthy pregnancy and avoid any risk to my unborn baby. I tried to reassure myself that in a few days time my scan would put my mind at rest, but a vague sense of impending disaster – an uneasiness in the back of my mind – remained with me throughout. Part of me felt vulnerable and just wanted to get home to "safety" and a normal routine. Another part of me told me not to be so silly, to think positively that all would be well. Altogether I felt uneasy but I tried not to show it. I didn't want to upset everyone else by "bleating" about my fears, and I wanted my husband to enjoy the week away. We hadn't had a holiday for a long time and I didn't want to spoil it, so I had a few firm words with myself and began to relax.

On the day of the scan, my bubble burst. I was told that although I had been pregnant, the baby was not developed. It was just an empty gestational sac – a blighted ovum. So, my doubts were confirmed. In a way I wasn't surprised because I had a feeling something was wrong, almost all along, so it wasn't so much of a shock than a depressing confrontation with the truth I knew inevitably awaited me. Nevertheless, it was no easier to bear and filled me with a desperate sadness. I felt devastated although it had, I have to admit, all seemed a little too good to be true. Thankfully, my husband is a great stabilizing force. His motto and favourite song is Monty Python's "Always look on the bright side of life" and he sings it as a reminder whenever I look downhearted! He is right of course. What will be will be, and life is too short to spend it dwelling on negativity or mourning what might have been.

However, positive thinking is hard work! For me it came in fits and starts. I could talk myself into seeing things philosophically whilst at home with my husband or when I had a chance to be alone with my thoughts, but I knew that I had an emotional struggle on my hands. You see, a close friend of mine became pregnant at the same time – in fact we conceived within a few days of each other. At the time, of course, it was tremendously exciting because it meant that we would be "growing" together, attending ante-natal classes, clinics etc., together, and would be able to share the entire experience. It was her first pregnancy too, and until then she was my only close friend who, like me, had yet to start a family. It gave me a sense of security knowing that I wasn't alone, and felt time was still on my side so long as someone else was still in the race with me. When we became pregnant simultaneously therefore, it couldn't have been better, because it meant that neither of us would be left behind. When my own pregnancy came to an end, I found it very hard to cope with seeing Sandra every day, knowing that she still had her baby alive and well inside her. I was happy for her of course, but at the same time I couldn't shake off a most disturbing feeling. I felt I had been betrayed. I was angry at life for having cheated me out of my baby and I felt that my only ally had deserted me. I had been waiting for so long, surely I had reached the front of the queue. Surely it was my turn by now.

It was a ridiculous feeling and I hated myself for allowing such thoughts to get the better of me, but it ate away at me for days. I think it boiled down to the fact that I couldn't cope with the future, and all the old negative feelings kept flooding back. What if I never got pregnant? What if none of my eggs fertilized properly? What if this was the closest I would ever get? I felt as though I were stuck on a treadmill. Everything seemed so utterly bleak. I so desperately wanted a child and yet I knew that all those negative feelings were, in themselves, spoiling my chances.

I found myself going through spells of intense anguish. Something would remind me and then the tears would start again. Uncontrollable sometimes, but I felt much better for a good cry as it released the emotion. I kept thinking about the sheer bad luck of it all, about my friend Sandra and how good it was going to be. Then I would look at my flat and empty tummy and be crippled with heartache and longing. This would probably sound pathetic to some, but most people would not understand. One always imagines that it is going to be so easy, something that happens naturally like any other human function, but when it doesn't, it is absolutely soul destroying because there is nothing one can do. Fertile women really do not know how lucky they are.

I decided at last that I should take some Remedies. I should have done so much sooner, but I just didn't feel in the right frame of mind to even think about it. However, I mixed myself up a combination of **Star of Bethlehem** to help heal my grief, **Sweet Chestnut** because I felt so utterly forlorn and dejected, **Clematis** as this is my type remedy, and at the bottom of it all was the awful prospect of having nothing to look forward to, **Honeysuckle** for all the regrets and the "what might have been" syndrome, and **Willow** because without a doubt I was feeling resentful and bitter towards life and, I'm ashamed to say, towards Sandra for having joined "the club" without me. I was angry and envied everyone with a baby, and I hated God for being so cruel. I added **Holly** for this vehement emotion.

That little lot seemed to do the trick. At last I began feeling more like my old self and before long regained some semblence of a sense of humour which I thought I had lost forever. I felt I had climbed out of the dark rut – a ray of sunshine was entering my life again. I reminded myself that although I had no baby to show for it, I had conceived, and so I knew that I could at least get pregnant. I therefore started looking at this unfortunate and distressing incident as a real sign of hope that it would only be a matter of time before I conceived again. After all, my body knew what to do now and having done it once, surely it would do it again! I still feel sad at times however, and I'm still wrestling with a heaviness inside me as I see Sandra reaching the milestones, as her pregnancy develops, that I would have been reaching with her. When she caresses her swollen abdomen, or protectively rests her hands upon it, as all pregnant women seem to do, it is like a knife turning in an open wound, but day by day that wound seems to be healing. At times I find it hard to conceal my feelings, and I'm afraid this has upset Sandra too which I feel guilty about because for her it is a time of great joy and it is unfair to darken her happiness with my own sorrowful self pity. Fortunately we are able to talk about our feelings and therefore help each other which is important for us both as she has her own grief and sadness to cope with too, and of course, the Remedies help as well, and I do turn to them when I need to.

So . . . it's back to the drawing board, but at least this time we can feel secure in the knowledge that it **can** work, **has** worked and **will** work again. As my husband keeps saying "always look on the bright side of life", so we do, or at least try to, but one day our turn will come and then, who knows? It might even be twins!

I just wanted to thank you for all your help in the past, and to thank Dr. Bach for providing us with the Flower Remedies and thus the means to cope with such destructive feelings that come our way, growing at times like an emotional cancer. I really don't know how I would have got through it all without their help.

With love,

Jennifer."

> "Some things in life are bad
> They can really make you mad
> Other things just make you swear and curse.
> When you're chewing on life's gristle
> Don't grumble, give a whistle
> And this'll help things turn out for the best.
> So, Always look on the bright side of life
> Always look on the light side of life.
> If life seems jolly rotten,
> There's something you've forgotten,
> And that's to laugh and smile and dance and sing.
> When you're feeling in the dumps
> Don't be silly chumps,
> Just purse your lips and whistle, that's the thing,
> And always look on the bright side of life!"
>
> Eric Idle

CHAPTER SIX

Women In Society

I. WORK AND FAMILY

The role of women in society has changed considerably over the years. In the pre-war era and for some time beyond, women were generally regarded as housewives and mothers; their function being to look after house and home, clean, cook, and rear children. A woman at one time who wanted to work was frowned upon as someone too "flighty" to be a "decent" wife. This is why women were not, generally, given positions of responsibility, nor their career aspirations taken seriously. Employers assumed that they would get married, have children and leave the firm. Some employers refused to even take women on at all because they considered them to be too unreliable for this reason.

Thankfully, times changed and as women made more and more of a stand, and demanded equal opportunities to their male counterparts, more career prospects opened up for them. Although there is still a residual proportion of employers that have not moved forward, the Equal Pay Act and Sex Discrimination Act have cemented women's status in society. Schoolgirls are encouraged to think about their future career and what they wish to study at higher education in order to achieve the direction in which they wish to go, or encouraged to at least consider what they would like to do when they leave school. It is no longer only boys who are primed for the world of work. Marriage and families have become something to look ahead to – careers now tending to take precedence – and it is not at all unusual for women to pursue a career first and then settle down to marriage and children later on, sometimes not until their mid thirties, or even later. Even then, many women are eager to return to work and resume an active role outside the family as soon as possible. Others are happy to regard starting a family as a form of career change in itself and so become full-time mothers while their children grow up.

There are, however, a number of women who find themselves not only following a demanding career, but running a home and bringing up a young family as well. Some women are the main bread-winners and so their work becomes even more of a responsibility. This situation has the potential to be extremely stressful if the children are ill, for example, or the house is in need of repair. At times like this, everything begins to mount up, one's ability to cope comes into question, tension rises and tempers are easily ignited. **ELM** is a very helpful remedy should this series of events sound familiar. It is for people who are normally confident and capable, but when the pressure mounts or responsibility becomes overwhelming, they begin to lose that self assurance and become disillusioned with their apparent lack of ability to cope. **IMPATIENS** would also help tempers with short fuses, and **HOLLY** if there is much spiteful or explosive anger. **VERVAIN** is another important remedy for tension, and may be a type remedy for a number of career women whose perfectionistic and enthusiastic nature causes them to become frustrated when they are prevented from moving forward, and as a result become keyed up and find it hard to relax. Vervain people can be angered if they sense injustice or unfair treatment, and the remedy helps such people to wind down so that they are able to "switch off" and relax, both mentally and physically. **BEECH** would help those who find themselves criticizing and unable to tolerate what seems to them to be other people's stupidity. Again, this feeling can cause a lot of inner tension, and if it is due to intolerance, Beech is the remedy to help.

There are also women who find themselves not following a career or line of work they enjoy particularly, but doing it all the same because they have to, in order to stay afloat financially. Money, when it is in short supply, is probably one of the biggest sources of worry, and central to numerous fraught arguments and disharmony in the home. Unfortunately, the only thing that will really put the problem aright is financial security, and of course the Remedies are unable to do that (if only they could!), but they can certainly help people in this situation to cope with life's difficulties and be able to approach the problem more rationally, working together instead of against each other. **WHITE CHESTNUT** is the ideal remedy for worried minds. It helps to bring mental arguments and unwanted troublesome thoughts that tend to go round and round in circles to a halt, allowing the mind to be still and thus obtain much needed rest, and in turn promote clearer thought. **OLIVE**, being the remedy for tiredness, is also a beneficial remedy to bear in mind, because not only may there be disturbed sleep due to worry, but physically having to work, clean, cook, entertain, bath and clothe young children every day, when you have more than enough on your mind to cope with already, can be thoroughly exhausting.

Single mothers may find the above particularly relevant. Having only one income to live on can make life extremely difficult and worrying. Inevitably it can be a vicious circle because although a single mother needs to work to make money, if she has a young baby or pre-school child to look after, she either has to find a nursery or child-minder which presents a further financial burden, or seek the help of relatives or friends which is not always consistent and therefore cannot be relied upon. There are state nursery schools but places are notoriously few and far between and private nurseries can be expensive. Many single mothers, therefore, find themselves relying on state benefits until their child starts school. Firms that supply creche facilities help to ease the problem for women with young children enormously, because it removes their biggest obstacle, but unfortunately not many companies offer these facilities to their work-force. It is not uncommon, and is very understandable, for women in a situation like this to become depressed and resentful, perhaps hopeless of finding a suitable solution. **GENTIAN** will help relieve the despondency, **WILLOW** the resentment, and **GORSE** will restore hope. Those who feel utterly dejected would find **SWEET CHESTNUT** brings light back into their life and thoughts. **WHITE CHESTNUT** will help restore calm to a worried mind, **MIMULUS** and **ASPEN** for an apprehensive uneasiness, and **OLIVE** for exhaustion; all remedies to consider. In addition, if resignation or apathy sets in, then **WILD ROSE** will help to build enthusiasm, and **HORNBEAM** will give strength to those who find it hard to get up and face the day, or procrastinate over some job they know they should do. Not everyone, of course, is affected by negativity. Some plod on bravely and always look at things positively and rationally. These people are **OAK** types, and the remedy will help should that inner resilience and natural strength begin to wane. Those who **pretend** to be brave, and are always seen to be cheerful and "on top of things", but secretly, underneath, suffer agonizing worry, fear, lack of confidence or whatever, are **AGRIMONY** people, and their remedy will help to relieve all that inner torture. There may be other remedies that will help too, such as **LARCH** to restore confidence in oneself, and **ROCK WATER** for those who refuse to accept help as they consider taking advantage of a helping hand to be a sign of weakness, so they deny themselves the opportunity, should it come their way, of making life a little bit easier.

When children start school, it may come as a welcome relief to the woman who has struggled whilst they were very young, but generally, even bearing this in mind, it is a rather nostalgic time for a mother, as it marks the end of an era. Her child is growing up, becoming independent and will begin to develop his or her own individuality. It is therefore a time of adjustment, and for those who find it hard to get used to, **WALNUT** will help to make it easier. **HONEYSUCKLE** will help if you should feel nostalgic and allow your thoughts to linger so much on the memories of your child's first few years, that they become all-absorbing and distract you from enjoying the present stage of development. For those who find it hard to let go, perhaps fussing too much, **CHICORY** would help counter the desire to cling and thus allow the child's free spirit to grow and develop. For mothers who are over-anxious for their children, who worry and fear unduly for their well-being, and are unable to relax until the child is home safe and sound again, **RED CHESTNUT** will help.

In addition to helping you as a mother, the remedies are also there to help your children should they be needed. Starting school can be traumatic for the child, and the Remedies will help relieve anxieties from the young mind **MIMULUS** for the fear element, **ASPEN** for apprehension, **WALNUT** if he or she finds it hard to settle down, **CHICORY** if he clings and does not want to let go of the secure familiarity of mother and home, **ROCK ROSE** if there is terror, **CHERRY PLUM** for hysteria, loss of control or panic, or **RESCUE REMEDY** which would be more ideal as it would also offer the soothing properties of Star of Bethlehem in addition to those of Rock Rose and Cherry Plum. Helping your child to adapt in this way will also help you to relax and adjust so that you can progress through these transitional periods positively together.

Some women, whether they are mothers or not, suffer with considerable boredom. This is especially apparent if there is nothing else to occupy the mind other than home-life and housework. Women with young children frequently say that they long for an adult conversation; that they spend all day every day, talking only to children, and as a result feel that they are losing their own independence and individuality. For the boredom, **CLEMATIS** may help as at times like this, the mind often tends to drift into a fantasy of what might be, or what could be. If it causes you to be irritable or "niggly" with your children, then try **IMPATIENS** for the impatience and **BEECH** for the intolerance. You may also benefit from **SWEET CHESTNUT** if you feel you are locked into a routine and can see no way out. These remedies may also be helpful to housewives whose children have grown up and perhaps left home, and are feeling at a loose end – no longer having to take children to school, dress them, feed them, tidy up after them etc. This is when boredom can really set in, especially if no close friends live nearby. It can be all too easy to slip into an apathetic frame of mind and just drift. If you feel like this **WILD ROSE** is the remedy you need. For those who feel lethargic, as though they have little energy to face the day ahead, **HORNBEAM** will help the enthusiasm for living return. **MUSTARD** will help those who feel depressed for no particular reason, and feel there is little joy in life. For those whose husbands work away or are involved in a lot of travelling, **RED CHESTNUT** will help ease the fears of an over-anxious mind, should for example, they not return home on time.

II. LONELINESS

Dr. Bach catagorized his remedies into seven groups, and the fifth group is headed "loneliness", under which he listed three remedies: **WATER VIOLET, IMPATIENS** and **HEATHER**. Whilst these are not remedies for the feeling of loneliness per se, there are individual aspects of each which may apply, depending on your particular personality and nature. **WATER VIOLET** is for those who actually prefer their own company. They may choose to be solitary; may prefer to remain single, but whether they marry or not, they are private people; reserved. They tend to keep a "safe distance" from others, maybe even their husband or partner is not invited to know the Water Violet completely. As a couple, they may keep themselves to themselves, but there are many who marry more open and social men who tend to take on the "friendly neighbour" role, enabling the Water Violet to enjoy her privacy and quietude. People of this nature do not openly discuss their feelings with others and may feel lonely due to the solitary aspect of their personality. Other people may feel that it would be too much of an intrusion on the Water Violet's privacy to offer their friendship and so, sadly, and perhaps reluctantly, stay away. As a result, the Water Violet may feel even more isolated and instead of relishing the peace and solace of aloneness, she finds herself the victim of loneliness. Water Violet, being her type remedy, would help her to bridge the gap with the outside world so that others can see that she is not too proud or too self-contained to appreciate a little company from time to time.

HEATHER people, as a complete contrast, are those who are **very** social – they are talkative people and will, given the chance, tell you all about themselves, their family, friends, home, garden, work etc. Dr. Bach fondly called them "button-holers" because they tend to talk closely to your face to keep your attention. Heather people therefore feel lonely if they lose companionship – lose someone to talk to. It is then that the negative aspects of their nature becomes apparent because it is then that they "button-hole" anyone who comes along, anyone who will listen, and as a result, sadly, tend to be avoided which only exacerbates their loneliness. It therefore becomes a vicious circle. Heather will help such people to be able to realise that companionship is not a one-sided relationship, help them appreciate that listening to what other people have to say is more interesting than it may have once seemed, and this two-way participation is of mutual benefit and thus central to establishing a lasting friendship.

IMPATIENS people are those who are very quick of mind and action. They think, talk and move quickly. They are easily irritated with those who are slow and become impatient to finish a job or a sentence. They are often fidgety, eager for the next task, their mind racing ahead. Such people tend to work alone so that they can work at their own pace and not be hindered by others who are slow and methodical. This need for space and solitude is a trait of both Impatiens and Water Violet, but in quite different ways and for very different reasons. However, if the Impatiens, in her need for her own space, cuts herself off from others, perhaps even becoming bad tempered and impatient with them, then loneliness may result. For women of this nature, Impatiens is the remedy to help ease the lonely feelings, and help them take a little more time so that they can comfortably live and work with others, even those who are not as hasty as they, and thus enjoy the companionship that will then have a chance to develop.

The above is by no means a definitive list – people with quite different natures may suffer with loneliness. Always consider your individual feelings and your individuality in order to find the remedy that suits your own personal needs.

There are numerous reasons why a woman might find

herself alone or feeling lonely. Divorce, separation, widow-hood, husbands or partners who work away from home for long periods at a time, or go out on their own every evening, are all predisposing to loneliness. Similarly, the woman who lives alone by choice may also go through periods of feeling desperately lonely.

Living alone, however, can nevertheless be tremendously fulfilling, and remaining single can give a woman the free-dom to enjoy her independence free from the constraints of a marriage partnership. Being able to do what you please, when you please, make your home the way you want it, and be able to pursue the work and leisure activities you enjoy without having to concern yourself with the preferences of another individual, means you can think and live for your-self. There are some women, however, who find themselves alone, not by choice, but due to circumstances. Their thoughts may be tinged with rueful disappointment or regret because although one can enjoy the company of numerous friends and acquaintances, there is always the return home alone, and the quiet lonely nights without the comfort of someone to cuddle.

Adjustment is a major aspect of coping with solitude: Adjustment to a new way of life in the case of those who are divorced or separated, and adjustment to life as it is for those who find themselves on their own for other reasons. **WAL-NUT** is the remedy to help with this transition; to help you to settle into a new home environment or way of life; to help you move forward, free of the constraints of the past. Di-vorce or separation in itself can be most traumatic. There may be all kinds of reasons for the relationship breaking down, and so consequently the emotions that result can range from one extreme to the other. Many of the feelings associ-ated with grief may apply to circumstances of divorce – with the Bach Remedies, it is the mood or emotion that is the important factor, not the event that sparked it off. If there is guilt as a result of divorce, then **PINE** will apply in the same way as it would for a woman bereaved who reproaches herself. If you feel a deep despair and sense of loss then **STAR OF BETHLEHEM** and **SWEET CHESTNUT** would apply in the same way as they would if the cause was due to a bereavement. There may be a sense of resentment or bitterness which would require **WILLOW**, or **HOLLY** if the feeling is more vehement – hatred, jealousy or suspicion. The Remedies are there to help, and although cannot provide a different set of circumstances, they can help you to move forward with more hope and optimism and deal with the negative feelings that stand in the way of your enjoyment of life, replacing them with a more positive outlook towards a brighter future.

III. COPING WITH ILL-HEALTH

Dr. Bach believed that all disease originated as disharmony within our being – some blockage interfering with the flow of Life Force between spirit, mind and body. Disease, therefore, to Dr. Bach, was simply the manifestation of this disharmony; the body's way of expressing its dis-ease.

There are diseases and conditions with which we come into contact more and more frequently; diseases which did not seem to affect past generations – or perhaps they did, but had not at that time been given a definite label. Myalgic encephalomyelitis is one such disease. Irritable bowel syndrome is another. These, as well as others, such as thrush, affect men as well as women, but because there is a high incidence in the female population, we will consider each condition in turn.

Myalgic encephalomyelitis

This is more commonly known as "M.E." or "Post Viral Fatigue Syndrome" which is a descriptive title for the symptoms and occurrence of the disease. It follows a viral infection – influenza and glandular fever are two of the most common culprits. The initial viral disease apparently clears up, but the virus remains dormant in the system and from time to time revives itself to present periods of flu-like symptoms. Sometimes, these symptoms linger in constant succession, so that the system is never truly symptom-free. At one time, before it was completely understood, it was deemed to be "all in the mind" because the symptoms were so vague and no actual physical factor could be clearly identified. However, it is now accepted by most medical practitioners to be a real disease with real symptoms, although there is still a proportion of sceptical physicians who do not believe it exists.

The symptoms of M.E. can vary in severity from one individual to another, but there is one classic symptom which seems to apply to all sufferers and that is tiredness. This can be so extreme in some cases, that the sufferer can physically only cope with a few hours of mobility each day, needing to take excessive periods of rest. Lethargy can also be a common symptom, as well as a general feeling of malaise. Some people suffer with extreme nervousness, panic attacks, depresson or lack of concentration, others with joint pain and headaches. Whatever the symptoms may be, the important factor as far as the Bach Remedies are concerned, is the personality and the emotional outlook of the individual sufferer. M.E. frequently affects women (and men) who have demanding jobs, who work under pressure or are in positions of responsibility, and who, as a result, work long hours and over-tax themselves. When a person of such a nature becomes ill, they are usually those who will return to work too early, or even go on working despite their illness, ignoring their body's need to rest and thus not giving themselves a chance to recover. The system then becomes over-tired and as a result protests by **insisting** it rests. M. E. can be so debilitating it certainly achieves that!

In order to choose the most appropriate remedies, you need to consider your particular nature, temperament and character as well as your moods and emotions, so that you can put how you **feel** into context with how you **are**. If you are a go-ahead person, a workaholic, always active, suffering with stress and tension due to frustration, then the remedy you need is **VERVAIN**. If you are a very quick-minded person who is hasty in action, always conscious of time and thus impatient to reach schedules, **IMPATIENS** would be the remedy for you. If you are the sort of person who does not get worked up, but takes things in your stride, plods on through thick and thin, not succumbing to set-backs or frustration, but calmly pressing ahead in a strong and solid way, then the remedy for your "type" would be **OAK**. If you are very strict with yourself, making yourself follow a set routine, demanding discipline of yourself and expecting similar high standards from others, then **ROCK WATER** would be your personal remedy.

These are examples of constitutional "type" remedies which help you regain inner poise and harmony. However, when things go wrong, or when you do not feel well, something that would normally not present a major problem, becomes pressurising or burdensome, and so other remedies to tackle these moods are helpful too. **OLIVE** for example, will help to ease, or at least take the edge off, the fatigue, although tiredness in this case is usually symptomatic – the result of overwork for example, so it is important to treat the cause as well. **HORNBEAM** would help if you feel lethargic and weary, unable to face work, feeling that it is all too much of an effort, and wishing you could put it off until a later date. **WHITE CHESTNUT** helps the thoughts and mental arguments circling incessantly round in the mind. **ROCK ROSE** is the remedy to help ease terrifying anxieties, **CHERRY PLUM** for thoughts which get out of control, making mountains out of molehills and imagining situations out of all proportion. **MUSTARD** will help to lift the depression which descends for no apparent reason, drifting over you like a dark cloud. **GENTIAN** is for the known depression, when you know **why** you feel low, **SWEET CHESTNUT** will help ease the despair if you feel helpless and cannot see any light in the darkness ahead. **GORSE** will restore hope to those who have lost faith in a cure. **WILD ROSE** will help those who feel resigned to their suffering. **CRAB APPLE** will help those who feel "ill" and the need to be cleansed. **LARCH** will restore self-confidence to those who have lost it. **CERATO** will restore faith and belief in oneself, and trust in one's intuition and wisdom. **ELM** will help those who find responsibility too great, too heavy a burden, and feel inadequate and unable to cope with it. **CLEMATIS** will aid concentration if your mind has a tendency to "wander".

You may also find it helpful to add some of your remedy, or even **RESCUE REMEDY** to your bath water (about 20 drops) as this often has a relaxing effect. An aromatherapy bath is also very relaxing at the end of the day. I find a bath with a few drops of Lavender essential oil very soothing.

Other ways to relax are to take up regular yoga which helps you to begin the day feeling fresher, and helps you to unwind at the end. Or treat yourself to an aromatherapy massage, or chiropractic session if you suffer with backache. Both are wonderfully rejuvenating.

Irritable bowel syndrome

This disease is readily accepted as stress related, but is also associated with constipation caused by a lack of fibre in the diet. It is a very painful and distressing condition affecting the passage of stools along the gut. The large bowel, or colon, has a natural peristaltic action – it contracts and relaxes along its length pushing the forming stool towards the rectum for expulsion. In irritable bowel syndrome, the stools tend to be hard and dry, giving rise to constipation. Constipation itself is not irritable bowel, but in those who suffer with this condition, the hard stool irritates the lining of the bowel, causing inflammation which is sore. In response to that, spasm of the bowel occurs, and together they cause intense pain. The pain is generally felt in the lower abdomen either on one side or the other, but more commonly on the left. It is a griping pain that comes in waves and can be excruciating at times. Emptying the bowel relieves the pain, but due to constipation and its residual irritation, it usually only gives temporary relief. Soon the pain will return as the bowel goes into further spasm as it tries to expel the bulky stool. Eventually the bowel will empty and the pain will go. As with M.E., the severity of irritable bowel varies from person to person. Some suffer with these bouts of pain once in a while, others suffer with almost constant pain.

Diet is obviously important. Eat plenty of green vegetables, fresh fruit and salad, and drink plenty of water and juice. Fibre too is extremely important in order to keep the stools soft and thus avoid irritation to the bowel lining. Wholemeal bread and cereal as well as green leafy vegetables are all good sources of fibre. Bran itself is rather tasteless on its own, but it does make a good thickener for certain dishes which makes it more acceptable. Some breakfast cereals such as "All-bran" provide an excellent supply of bran. Muesli cereals are also good fibre providers but are sometimes considered too "dry" and thought to aggravate the condition. However, if plenty of fluid is taken during the course of the day, it should overcome that particular problem.

Regular exercise is also important because this helps to increase the oxygen supply to all parts of the body and tones the system. Rather like a car's engine, we need to be taken for regular "runs" to maintain good working order! Yogic exercises are excellent for promoting good bowel action and are best performed first thing in the morning before taking any food or drink. Sit on the floor, cross-legged or in the lotus or half-lotus position, whichever is more comfortable, with the back straight, but not stiff. If you are used to yoga, you will appreciate the importance of beginning with some relaxing breathing exercises. Close your eyes, have your hands resting on your knees, palms upwards with the thumb and index finger touching. This is the yogic posture. Now, breath out, through your nose, empty your lungs, and then slowly breath in again through your nose, first filling your chest, allowing your shoulders to rise as your chest expands, then as your breath becomes deeper, push your abdomen out. When you have taken as deep a breath as you can, slowly begin breathing out again, through your nose, allowing your shoulders to relax and drawing your abdomen in. Repeat this complete breath a few times, but do not strain. Then, you can begin your bowel exercises. Remain seated in the same posture and breath normally. Place your hands on your lower abdomen and contract your abdominal muscles. Now release them. Contract them again, and then this time, push them out more forcefully. "Snap" them out. Contract in, snap out. Do this three or four times quite quickly at about ½–1 second intervals. Now relax, and breath normally. Take a complete, deep breath as above, and then do the bowel exercise again, working up to 10 contractions. Then rest again, breath normally, and then complete your routine with a complete breath. This bowel exercise encourages the stimulation of peristalsis and maintains healthy bowel movement.

An attack of irritable bowel tends to occur when the sufferer is going through an upsetting or tiring period, or has more than a usual amount of responsibility or worry. Avoidance of stress, therefore, and a gentle means of dealing with it when it does occur, is naturally the best way to approach the problem, prevention always being far better than cure. In addition to the above practical suggestions, the Bach Remedies will also help you to relax and keep your mind calm. Similar remedies that were discussed in the section about M.E. will also apply to irritable bowel because similar factors are pre-disposing to both conditions. **VERVAIN** for the workaholic; **IMPATIENS** for irritability, impatience and the stress of working to deadlines; **WHITE CHESTNUT** for worrying thoughts; **OLIVE** for tiredness and exhaustion; **ASPEN** for apprehension and feeling always "on edge"; **BEECH** for feeling "niggly" and critical; **WILLOW** for resentment or self-pity which is a common repercussion of too much responsibility and pressure – "nobody understands what it is like"; **SWEET CHESTNUT** for despair – crying in desperation; **ELM** for responsibility that gets too much to cope with, and **RESCUE REMEDY** for emergencies, when you are in pain or feel in a state of shock or panic.

In addition, consider your character and natural temperament, and choose remedies that apply to your personality type.

Relieving tension through exercise and relaxation

Aromatherapy, massage and chiropractic are all helpful ways of releasing tension, but for something that you can easily do yourself, deep relaxation exercises and meditation are excellent ways of regaining peace and inner quiet. If you can relax completely for 10 minutes each day, you will find that sleep is more refreshing and you are thus better prepared for the next busy day. Find some time to yourself, when you can be alone and undisturbed (easier said than done I know!). Wear something loose and comfortable, and lie down on a firm mattress or on the floor. Lie on your back, with your palms uppermost, arms a few inches away from your sides, and your legs slightly apart. Now, close your eyes, and try to picture your body as it lies on the floor. Then, focus your attention on each part of your body in turn, starting with your feet, working up your legs, along the length of your trunk, to your shoulders, down your arms to your fingers, then your neck and face. As you picture each part of your body, tense the muscles in that area. Really work them, extend and contract the muscles. Hold for a few seconds then gradually release the tension and allow that area to relax again, but this time concentrate on the relaxation. Gradually work your way over your whole body in this way, tensing and then relaxing each part. When you have finished, cast your mind's eye over your entire body, and notice any parts that are not completely limp. Relax them, let your body sag, allow your mouth to fall open and your breathing to become shallow. Let your mind drift towards a calming thought – picture a place that you like, or a flower or a painting that appeals to you, or imagine yourself in the sun, on a beach, far away from the hustle and bustle of work and daily routine. Try to maintain this tranquility for as long as you can, but even if you only manage it for a few minutes you will feel so much better for it.

Exercise generally is a good way of getting rid of excess adrenalin, built up during a trying day at work. It helps to relieve anger and frustration too, and if you are feeling tired or "muggy", aerobic exercise such as running, jogging, cycling, swimming or "aerobics" will help to replenish your energy. Running and cycling are not everybody's idea of fun, although cycling can be used purposefully, to get to work for example, which then makes it an excellent way to obtain regular exercise as well as providing you with a means of transportation. Exercise, however, should be enjoyed. It should not become another chore that you **have** to do and would rather not. If you can enjoy it then you will want to do it regularly and that is what you are trying to achieve. Swimming, for most people, is relaxing as well as good exercise, and although it involves travelling to the swimming pool at a time which is not always convenient, and getting changed into a costume which, in the middle of winter, is not so appealing, it is nevertheless a worthwhile activity because you feel so "alive" and toned up at the end of a session. It is also a means of exercising muscles that other exercises do not reach – the water suspends the body, removing the strain of its weight, and thus allows excellent toning to take place whilst the whole body is supported. Other activity sports such as tennis and squash are also extremely good aerobic sports, and so if this is something that you find more appealing and you have a partner who would also like to keep fit, then this may well prove to be ideal for you both. If, however, the above action sports all sound too energetic, a simple brisk walk will do a power of good.

For relaxation, it is a matter of finding what is right for you. If you enjoy painting, this makes an excellent way to relax – your mind is focused on what you are doing and the actual act of drawing the brush across paper in gentle strokes is calming in itself. Knitting and sewing can also be just as effective. So too is listening to, or playing music. It is a matter of choosing the activity that you enjoy – something that you can get "lost" in. Gardening is also a very good way to relax, and is good exercise too. For those who are keen gardeners, this may be the ideal solution, and for those of you who are not, it may generate an interest. Gardening need not be strenuous and does not always have to involve digging and mowing. Container gardening is equally enjoyable and rewarding, especially if you have grown your plants from seed; you can really enjoy the fruits of your labours and feel a good sense of achievement and job satisfaction! Even ironing **can** be relaxing – difficult to believe, but nevertheless true! It allows you to think, lets your mind drift and daydream while your hands automatically run the iron over endless shirts, tea-towels, and maybe, even the odd item of sports gear!

Thrush

Candida Albicans, commonly known as "thrush", is a fungal yeast infection affecting the sexual organs. It develops in the vagina where and when the conditions for it are right, and causes intense itching and soreness together with a vaginal discharge which resembles cottage cheese. It tends to occur when the sufferer is at a low ebb, or under stress, and is, unfortunately a very common complaint, and those who suffer with it, usually find that it returns again and again. There are some aggravating factors besides tiredness, depression, ill-health or stress, and these include excess heat and sweatiness, during warm weather for example, or long-distance travelling, especially in a hot climate, or due to wearing tight clothing, or pants made from synthetic material. Not everyone suffers with it, and so not everyone who happens to wear synthetic knickers, for example, will be affected, just as there are many people who can walk through long grass without suffering with hay fever. However, if you are troubled, then Remedies to choose would be those that treat the pre-disposing factors such as the tiredness or stress, but you may also find that bathing the area with a cool solution of water containing a few drops of **Rescue Remedy** and **Crab Apple** very soothing. **Rescue Remedy Cream** may also be helpful and perhaps an application of this at night, around the entrance to your vagina will help to ease the irritation and thus enable the inflammation and soreness to die down.

Sexually Transmitted Disease

There are numerous sexually transmitted diseases, and I feel it would be helpful to mention some of them briefly here as they do affect social activity.

Gonorrhoea and Syphilis are the "classic" STD's. Gonorrhoea is more common than syphilis and is highly infectious on sexual contact with an infected partner. It can be passed from man to woman or woman to man, and once transmitted to a woman, lives in the warm moist atmosphere of the vagina. The symptoms of gonorrhoea are an unusual, creamy yellow vaginal discharge, burning when passing water, and sometimes abdominal discomfort. However, in the **MAJORITY** of women, no symptoms occur at all, and so a woman may be unaware that she has the disease, and may only become suspicious when her partner complains of symptoms. The danger of undiagnosed gonorrhoea is ascending infection to the uterus and Fallopian tubes which may cause salpingitis (inflammation of the tubes), and subsequent infertility. However, the disease is curable and the complications can be avoided by early diagnosis and treatment. It is therefore wise to have a check-up if you are at all concerned about the possibility of having contracted the disease.

Syphilis is less common but is a dangerous disease. It can have long term complications affecting the nervous system and the heart if left untreated. The first stage of syphilis is a painless sore appearing on the sex organs – and sometimes this occurs inside the vagina where it is unseen, and because it is painless, may not be noticed. The second stage is a body rash of pink spots and a general feeling of malaise. The rash lasts several weeks. Stage three of the disease is a dormant period when it seems to have disappeared. However, it remains present in the body and at some time in the future may be re-activated and cause serious nervous disorders and/or damage to the heart, eyes and ears. If it is diagnosed before this occurs, however, the disease is completely curable.

Herpes has been given a great deal of publicity in recent years, generating a degree of fear and hopelessness in those suffering with this disease. There are five strains of the virus – chicken pox, glandular fever, cytomegalovirus, Herpes Simplex Virus 1 and Herpes Simplex Virus 2. Herpes Virus 1 affects the lips causing a sore to appear, commonly known as a cold sore. Herpes Virus 2 is the strain affecting the genitals. Although Herpes Virus 1 **can** be spread to cause genital herpes it does not mean that a cold sore has been sexually transmitted. There are many people who suffer with cold sores who have never had or been in contact with any form of genital disease. It is, however, infectious and because it affects the mucus membrane, can infect the genitals if contact takes place whilst a sore is active and open. It is therefore important to avoid self-infection by taking care of personal hygiene and always making sure you have washed your hands immediately after touching your lip. Cold sores often appear due to stress or an unsettled period, and can also be aggravated by the sun. Some people have found that an application of **Rescue Remedy Cream** to the sore as soon as it begins to appear has helped the pain to subside and allowed healing to begin, resulting in a less severe attack.

The signs of Herpes Virus 2 are a cluster of blisters on the genitals which burst and then scab over. When the scab falls away or is knocked off, the sore underneath is highly infectious. It is an extremely painful condition and may necessitate the use of pain-killers. Friction and moisture encourage the disease to spread and so the vulva should be kept clean and dry – easier said than done, but wearing loose cotton pants, like French Knickers can help. Although not a treatment for the Herpes Virus itself, **Rescue Remedy Cream** may help to relieve the discomfort of genital herpes, or you may prefer to try a lotion of water containing a few drops of both Rescue Remedy and **Crab Apple** to gently bathe the area.

Due to a great deal of publicity, Herpes 2 has earned itself a reputation of being an incurable and painful disease that will return again and again for ever. Whilst this is, to some extent, true, the virus tends to attack only a few times in women and the first attack is the worst, secondary and recurrent attacks being less severe. Some women may never have a recurrence. There is, however, a lot of emotional upset that goes with the diagnosis of herpes – despair, depression, shock, guilt and fear – and although the Bach Remedies are not a cure for Herpes itself, they can help to reduce the emotional anguish. **GENTIAN** for the depression, or **SWEET CHESTNUT** if the outlook generally seems bleak; **STAR OF BETH-LEHEM** for the shock of the diagnosis; **PINE** if you feel guilty for having contracted it or passed it on to your partner; **MIMULUS** for fear, or **ROCK ROSE** for terror and panic. Although it is a sexually transmitted disease, Herpes Simplex Virus 2 is not classified as a "venereal disease" under the 1917 Venereal Diseases Act which only included gonorrhoea, syphilis and "soft sore". It should not, therefore, carry the stigma that has been attached to these other diseases which are generally associated with promiscuity. The Herpes virus can be passed on at birth from a mother with the disease to her child, and so it may lie dormant in your system all your life, until it is activated for one reason or another. It does not, therefore, relate to promiscuity – indeed you may suffer with it even if you have only had one partner. Any sexually transmitted disease, however, so often causes a sense of self-disgust, or uncleanliness for which **CRAB APPLE** is the ideal remedy, helping to relieve these self-condemning emotions.

Since AIDS has become a well-publicised disease, the use of condoms as a means of protection against transmission has been encouraged. Condoms went out of favour at one time because they were a nuisance and rather a cumbersome intrusion into one's enjoyment of spontaneous sex. However, they have benefits which are not found in any other contraceptive device, in that they provide an almost complete barrier between the male and female genitalia, and thus considerably reduce the risk of contracting any sexually transmitted disease.

Any sexual activity, but especially with a new partner, carries with it the fear associated with "catching something". AIDS is currently the most feared disease because it is so life threatening, but whatever the object of the fear, the fear itself is the factor of significance when considering the Bach Remedies. **MIMULUS** is the obvious choice for any known fear, or **ROCK ROSE** for terror. However, the fear may not be for your own health and safety, but for that of someone you love in which case the remedy **RED CHESTNUT** would be more appropriate.

AIDS itself has been given a lot of media coverage. There are still many unanswered questions, but it is being understood more and more all the time. However, despite all the publicity, there is also a great deal of ignorance and confusion. It **may** be passed on by sexual activity, but it need not be. Similarly, it **may** be caused by sharing an infected needle for injection, but it need not be. It can just as easily be spread through blood transfusion by using blood from an infected donor, or by accident should any blood to blood contact be made. Stringent tests are carried out on all blood taken from donors, but there have been reported incidents when an infected sample has got through undetected. It can, therefore, affect anyone and is not confined to the sexually promiscuous, drug addicts or homosexual men as is often thought, wrongly, to be the case.

Fear is one element of the virulent nature of AIDS, but for someone suffering with it, the emotional strain may take any form, ranging from utter despair and hopelessness to a complacent resignation. Any of the 38 Remedies may therefore be required, and of course, the type of person concerned is an important consideration and a remedy descriptive of the character should also be included. For hopelessness and a bleak pessimism, **GORSE** is the remedy to restore hope; **WILD ROSE** will help those who are apathetic or resigned to whatever lies in their path. **AGRIMONY** will help those who appear to be cheerful, carefree and in control on the surface, but hide their inner worries behind that facade.

OAK is for those who struggle on bravely trying anything and everything, never giving up hope of finding a cure, yet may **over-**do it and begin to lose their inner strength and perseverence. **OLIVE** will help those who are tired and weakened through exhaustion; **HORNBEAM** for those who need strength to face each day. **WHITE CHESTNUT** is the remedy to help combat the whirlpool of thoughts; **ASPEN** for the apprehensive feeling of "something" being about to happen; **HOLLY** for those who feel they hate the world, hate God, hate what has happened to them; **WILLOW** for those who have a more festering grudge or sense of resentment or self-absorbed pity. **PINE** will help those who feel guilty, perhaps for being ill and letting their loved ones down – a natural feeling, despite there being no grounds for inflicting such blame on oneself. **CRAB APPLE** is the remedy to help those who dislike themselves or condemn themselves, unable to bear the sight of their own reflection.

As with any other condition or dis-ease, the Bach Remedies treat the moods and emotions; the personality and temperament. This, to Dr. Bach was the fundamental basis of all illness, and so his remedies are aimed at treating the cause rather than the effect. In selecting remedies therefore, one needs to put the condition to one side and concentrate wholly on the person as an individual for their own personal moods and emotional outlook, and for their individuality and uniqueness. Every one of us is different, and so different remedies will apply even though we may suffer with the same problem. The Bach Remedies are not designed to be a cure or treatment for physical complaints or medical conditions, and although they help promote the body's own disease-fighting mechanism, the body itself may not always be successful in eradicating a disease that has caused too much damage or taken too strong a hold. However, a diseased body is not a diseased soul, and so whatever the outcome, the Remedies are there to comfort the soul and the mind – the being as a whole – to reassure and calm so that life becomes more tolerable, happier and has a deeper and more meaningful sense of purpose.

"Nor need any case despair, however severe,
for the fact that the individual is still
granted physical life indicates that the
Soul who rules is not without hope."

Edward Bach, Heal Thyself.

IV. DIFFICULTIES WITH SEX

Although extremes, frigidity and frustration are probably the most commonly upsetting problems of a psycho-sexual nature that a woman will encounter. Ironically, frustration may eventually result in frigidity and similarly frigidity may eventually result in frustration, and so although these two conditions seem, at first, to be at opposite ends of the spectrum, they may be interlinked.

The word "frigidity" has a certain stigma attached to it and is a rather cumbersome word that often instils in one's mind a picture of a woman who cannot bear a man to touch her; someone who is cold and unlovable, or extremely "prim and proper" and who has a major sexual hang-up. This is, however, not what the word means at all. The correct term is "orgasmic dysfunction" meaning the inability for a woman to reach a climax. She may, therefore, be enjoying a perfectly normal loving relationship with her partner, she may even be having an enjoyable sex life, but is unable to reach an orgasm and is thus left feeling dissatisfied and increasingly saddened and worried by the condition.

Orgasm is achieved by physical stimulation of the clitoris and vagina, and because of this, it is often assumed that the inability to achieve an orgasm is due to some physical abnormality. This is, however, a misunderstanding, and although for a few women a physical disability may exist, for the majority the problem is of an emotional origin. Another common misconception is the confusion between being frigid and suffering with a condition called "vaginismus". This is a term which is given to women whose vaginal muscles go into spasm when sexual contact is made. Not only does it occur due to male approaches, but also to examination by a doctor. Even attempts to insert a tampon may set it off.

Difficulties with sex may be due to a number of things, but frequently they are based on fear: a rigid and highly disciplined or inhibited upbringing, for example, based upon an idea that sex is in some way "dirty"; having been frightened by what has been heard as a child; unpleasant memories of having been witness to parents' insensitive sexual activities. To a young child, seeing their parents making love, albeit accidentally, or a parent in the act with another man or woman, or witnessing an older sibling with a boyfriend or girlfriend in an uncompromising position can be a very frightening sight indeed, especially when the child has been brought up to believe that sex is a violation, or been provided with no sexual explanations. Frequently these children grow up harbouring a fear of sex all their lives, much disturbed by their childhood memories or experiences, and vowing never to allow a man to "attack" them like that. Gentle explanation at the time goes a long way to reassuring the young mind that there is nothing to fear; that it is something men and women who love each other do to express their love, that it is not painful or violent, and that "daddy" was not hurting "mummy". Unfortunately, there are a number of children who do grow up in fear and dread of it happening to them, perhaps having repeated nightmares, re-living the horror of what they have seen.

Other reasons may be based on ignorance. For example, if a girl is unprepared and has never seen an erect penis before, she might be terrified that it will not fit into her vagina, and so find the whole experience extremely upsetting. There may also be fear connected with the consequences of sexual activity – pregnancy, AIDS, sexually transmitted disease – or associated with actual penetration – fear of pain or trauma. Ignorance of anatomy may also cause fear and worry and result in tension. As far as the Bach Remedies are concerned, it is not what the woman is afraid *of* that matters, but just the simple fact that she *is* afraid.

Psycho-sexual problems such as these may take time and patience to put right, but with the help of the Remedies the process should be eased considerably. It would also be helpful to consider consulting a psycho-sexual counsellor – someone experienced in dealing sympathetically and impartially with such matters. There are nurses who have undergone special training in this field, often attached to family planning or specialised clinics. There are also trained counsellors who specialise in dealing with people who have personal difficulties. Help is also available through Marriage Guidance counselling.

Some useful addresses will be found at the back of the book.

Any difficulty, but especially sexual difficulties, inevitably put a strain on a marriage or partnership. The result may be tension, resentment and endless rows, but equally it may cause a gradual drifting apart, and when a relationship develops a "crack" like this, a lot of loneliness can soon fill the gap; feeling unloved, shunned, unattractive; out in the cold. If it goes on too long, a couple may need to get to know each other all over again, and so to repair the damage early is obviously important.

A woman's sexual difficulties may be compounded or even caused by her partner's own difficulties. Sexual incompetence in the male can certainly put a strain on a woman's own needs. Impotence and premature ejaculation are the most common male problems and although there are always a few exceptions, these conditions are also more often than not of an emotional origin. If a man reaches a climax too soon, it frequently means that insufficient time is available for the woman to be sufficiently aroused. Similarly, impotence leaves both partners feeling frustrated, but in addition to this, the man is left feeling inadequate, depressed that he is unable to perform the most basic function and therefore worried about his virility. He feels incomplete as a man for not being able to make love to his wife, and this in turn will inevitably cause problems for her. She may blame herself, worrying that her husband finds her unattractive or unsexy. Why does she not turn him on any more? Has he found someone else? Does he find her repulsive, fat or old and sagging? The emotional whirlpool has started and it is all too easy to be engulfed by the strength of its pull. Thankfully, the Remedies are there to help with the emotional aspects, but it is always easier to correct the problem at the outset than it is to leave it until it gets to this stage.

A couple who are under pressure due to responsibility, worry or problems with work, finance or family, may encounter sexual difficulties as a result of the frustration and tension that already exists. It may be responsible for sexual problems in the man, woman or both – stress and fatigue lowering the sexual drive or frustrating satisfaction – and so even in a loving relationship, a healthy sex life may not flourish. Pyscho-sexual problems are therefore circular, like a chain, and one thing will lead to another unless it is checked and corrected, thus breaking the chain reaction.

Libido is the manifestation of the sexual drive, and so lack of libido is a lack of sexual desire. It is commonly interpreted as frigidity, which although not strictly true, may be considered to be an off-shoot – being either the result of or a primary causal factor. It is quite normal for a temporary loss of sexual interest to occur during pregnancy, and it is common to find a pattern of greater and lesser desire occurring during the course of the menstrual cycle. It is also very common for libido to diminish when tired or under strain. However, if a woman is unable to enjoy sex, whatever the reasons may be, she may start to lose interest in it altogether. If it is not fulfilling, then why bother? Remedies in this situation once again should be based on the cause of the problem, but because apathy and resignation to the way things are can soon take over, the relationship may be in danger of going stale without having had the chance to remove the obstruction to a more enjoyable and satisfying life. This "stalemate" calls for **WILD ROSE** which is the remedy to bring excitement back into focus – to climb out of the rut of stagnation towards a more motivated and positive approach to bringing sex back to life. The submissive "lie back and think of England" approach to sex also calls for **WILD ROSE**, or **CENTAURY** if it is as a result of partner dominance. If the lack of libido is due to exhaustion, **OLIVE** would be helpful. **HORNBEAM** also assists in the revival of flagging enthusiasm and weariness – the "oh, can't it wait until morning" syndrome!

Because any problem related to sex affects both partners, it is always preferable to seek help together, recognizing that it is a problem you share. Difficulties encountered by the female as well as those encountered by the male are inextricably inter-linked and so in order to treat the root cause, both the man and the woman need careful counselling and guidance to enable them to understand each other's difficulties and how they can help one another to overcome them. Practical explanation providing frank advice of how to make mutual love-making really work is one aspect of beginning to build a fulfilling and complete relationship, but the basic cause needs to be tackled as well – the fear, anxiety, shock, horror, disgust or whatever it was that triggered the problem off in the first place. This is where the Bach Remedies can help, and will work hand-in-hand with the practical therapy and counselling. We are all individuals and so our needs differ. The personality of the person concerned is the key to their emotional balance and so the type remedy/ies should certainly be included. In addition to this, however, other remedies for the specific moods should be included as well, depending on individual needs. Remedies for emotions that have been discussed in this section are as follows:

STAR OF BETHLEHEM – for shock. This may be due to an experience in childhood, or due to the trauma and surprise of a sexual encounter in adult life.

ROCK ROSE – for terror.

CRAB APPLE – for a sense of disgust or contamination.

MIMULUS – for fear. This may be of sex, or even fear of the counselling session itself.

LARCH – self consciousness and fear of failure, or of giving an unsatisfactory performance.

AGRIMONY – for those who try to hide their fear, put on an act and pretend all is well.

WHITE CHESTNUT – for mental arguments, troublesome worrying thoughts.

HONEYSUCKLE – for re-living memories of some past event; haunting thoughts of a traumatic sight or sound.

WATER VIOLET – for those who are reserved and private; to help break the barriers of inhibition.

ROCK WATER – for those with a strict sense of duty, or who have been the victims of too rigid an up-bringing and as a result find themselves responding in a tense and rigid manner.

CENTAURY – for those who find themselves at the mercy of another; too weak to stand up for their own needs; find themselves victims of a dominant father or husband.

CHESTNUT BUD – to help one learn from past experience if the same situation arises time and again.

WILLOW – for resentment and bitterness towards parents, circumstances, life in general, or resentment towards a husband or partner who is unable to satisfy your needs.

HOLLY – for the anger that stems from envy, jealousy or hatred; perhaps even revenge and the desire to be destructive.

CHERRY PLUM – for irrational thoughts; ideas that get carried away, blowing things up out of all proportion.

WILD ROSE – for resignation.

HORNBEAM – if the thought of sex is a burdensome hurdle instead of a pleasure.

OLIVE – for fatigue.

BEECH – for intolerance of one's partner's "short-comings".

Relaxation tapes and yoga exercises are also excellent means of giving the mind and body a chance to unwind.

Physical exercise can also be extremely helpful as a means of releasing frustration and tension. It is healthy both for the mind and the body and allows the river of lively energy to flow throughout the whole being.

Another aspect to some relationship problems, is the need to hold on; to own or possess one's partner. This may stem from having been deprived of a stable relationship in the past, resulting in fear of being alone and thus desperately clinging to what love and stability there is. It can be highly counter-productive as overpowering eagerness for a relationship to work may be the very thing that brings it to an end; a greed for love can so easily turn to possessiveness, selfishness, suspicion and jealousy. To be emotionally bound and gagged in this way just creates tension in the relationship. Arguments begin, bad feeling develops and before long the rot sets in and marks the beginning of the end. Selfish love of this kind, and the lack of mutual understanding, care and respect for each other's needs, will undoubtedly put a strain on the sexual side of the relationship, if not the relationship itself. For it to work, there has to be give and take, so when one party does all the taking, anxious to satisfy his or her needs alone, then that essential mutual bond simply is not there and the whole thing inevitably collapses. The remedy for this negatively charged love is **CHICORY**, and the remedy will help to channel the need for love in a more positive and constructive way, thus allowing the other person the freedom they are entitled to; giving them room to breath. This in itself will relax the pent-up tension so that a warm and healthy glow can return. For those who are on the receiving end – for those who feel they are being stifled, **CENTAURY** will provide the strength to stand up for your **own** needs, and **WALNUT** will provide protection from the overpowering influence of your partner.

Whenever one discusses sexual problems, or when one worries about having a problem oneself, there is a temptation to question what is "normal". In fact, believing one is not normal because one's own body, habits or relationship do not seem to conform to those of others, or to the picture por-trayed by the media, allows depressing concern to set in that one may be considered abnormal or unacceptable, by the world at large. If you have nothing to compare your own experiences with other than what you have seen in films or on television, then it is quite understandable that you might feel your own relationship is lacking something, and so begin to worry about personal inadequacies. However, what you hear, read or see, or indeed learn from friends, can be terribly disconcerting and confusing when seeking some form of reassurance. Experience of previous relationships can also affect one's pre-conceptions and expectations of the next. What is "normal" can vary so much that there is really no accurate measurement. Essentially, it is what is right for **you**, with **your** partner, at a given time. The range of normality is vast, and attempting to determine what is normal in love and sex is like attempting to standardize hair or eye colour. Sexual fulfilment therefore is not something to which a yardstick approach can be applied. What one couple find unfulfilling may be another couple's joy. There are many women who worry because they have not experienced an orgasm, and yet might be enjoying a loving and satisfying relationship, and have been unconcerned until it was brought to the attention by a magazine article or conversation with a friend. Indeed, sexual climax is not the be-all and end-all by any means. In a tender stable relationship, sex can be just as fulfilling with or without the ultimate conclusion, although to achieve it will undoubtedly make it even better. Sometimes it just takes time, and I doubt if any woman experienced an orgasm the first time she made love. It is something that just happens, and may take practise to perfect – time to work out just how to make it happen – and this involves a gentle understanding of each other's needs. If that can be achieved, especially within a secure and warm loving relationship, it will, one day, happen unexpectedly – so just relax and allow nature to take its course.

CHAPTER SEVEN

SCREENING

THE CERVICAL SMEAR TEST

Of all screening procedures, this is the one most women should be familiar with. It is offered to all women once they have become sexually active, via their GP, Health Centre or Family Planning Clinic. Some areas have special Well Women Clinics which provide screening and advice for women of all ages.

Cervical cancer is a dangerous disease. It can spread quickly to the uterus and pelvis, affecting the ovaries, bowel, bladder and spine in its later stages. It is therefore vital to make an early diagnosis if it is to be treated successfully. In days gone by before the smear test was available, diagnosis was based on the symptoms a woman complained of, but this was most unsatisfactory because the disease is virtually asymptomatic in its early stages and so by the time a woman noticed changes in her vaginal discharge, experienced pain or irregular bleeding, it was often too late. Even surgery only prolonged life for a short time because of the highly invasive nature of this particular cancer. Thankfully the means of detecting the pre-cancerous changes in the cells of the cervix was discovered in 1943 by G. N. Papanicolau and H. E. Traunt, and their technique was further sophisticated by Ayre who introduced the use of a simple wooden spatula to scrape the cells from the cervix, which are then inspected under a microscope, and any abnormal cells or cell changes can be identified.

This was a tremendous breakthrough because it meant that early signs of cancer could not only be detected but treated, thereby preventing the development of the disease. In those early days, treatment was performed either by surgery or radiotherapy, but the development of more sophisticated micro-surgery techniques meant that surgical removal, if the disease was detected early enough, could be carried out by removing only the affected segment of the cervix – an operation called "cone biopsy" – thus overcoming the obvious disadvantages of more radical surgery. Radiotherapy too had its distinct contra-indications and side effects. The dangers of high-dose X-ray to the pelvis of a woman of childbearing age could have disastrous consequences on her fertility. So the development of laser technology, introduced into a few centres in the UK in the early 1980's, marked a major step forward. Not only was it simple to perform, destroying only the unhealthy cells and not harming any healthy tissue, it was also extremely successful – so much so, that early pre-cancerous lesions of the cervix are virtually certain of complete cure.

However, despite the success of the treatment, women were still presenting in much later stages of the disease, and consequently the death rate from cervical cancer continued to increase. Early detection through cervical cancer screening, therefore, is vital if we are to see an improvement in that pattern. Unfortunately despite health education programmes and public information, there remains a significant proportion of women who are reluctant to come forward. Reasons for this must be either ignorance of the test itself or its value, or because of fear. Certainly "cancer" is a frightening word and so to volunteer for a test that has the potential to diagnose it, naturally causes some apprehension. However, its diagnosis later on when the disease has had a chance to really establish itself, would be infinitely more frightening because the chances of cure would, by then, be seriously reduced. Indeed, early detection need not **BE** frightening because there is now a highly successful, safe and simple treatment, and a cure virtually guaranteed. It is important to stress that the earlier it is discovered, the better the chances of successful cure and so I urge every woman who is sexually active to go along for this quick and painless test. A few minutes out of your day to visit your doctor or clinic could save your life.

What does the screening test involve?

It is a very simple test which takes only a few minutes to perform. The doctor or nurse needs to wipe a small wooden spatula across the cervical opening in order to collect a smear of cells. To enable her to do so, she needs to be able to see your cervix and this means that an instrument called a speculum is inserted into your vagina to hold its walls apart. The speculum itself is rather a cumbersome object and looks a lot more awesome than it really is. Some are made of metal which, if not warmed beforehand, are rather cold; others are plastic which tend to be a little more comfortable in this respect. Although it might look as though it is going to be painful it really does not hurt at all. Once the speculum has been adjusted the nurse will be able to see your cervix clearly. She then shines a light along its length and takes the scraping she needs. This part of the test is also painless, although it is a peculiar sensation and may therefore feel a little uncomfortable. However, it is soon over – as I said, it literally takes only a minute or two. The smear is placed on a glass slide and sent to the laboratory. Probably the worst part of the entire procedure is waiting for the results! Unfortunately they can take a few weeks to come through, sometimes longer, and generally you will be told that you will only be informed if there is a problem. However, you will always be invited to ask for the result, when it is available to set your mind at rest.

The test should be repeated at regular intervals and depending on the area in which you live, this could be anything from two to five yearly. Once you have been screened, most centres have a re-call system so that you are contacted automatically when your next smear is due. However, it is a good policy to keep a record yourself so that you can make your own appointment when the time comes, just in case the re-call system fails, but having taken that important step to safeguard your health, you can relax in the interim, secure in the knowledge that all is well.

What happens if the test result is positive?

First of all, it should be emphasized that a positive result does not, in itself, mean you have cancer. The object of the smear test is to detect **PRE**-cancer cells. There are, nevertheless, varying degrees of pre-cancer cells, just as there are varying degrees of cancer itself. Treatment therefore, depends on the developmental stage. The mildest change in pattern is described as "dysplasia", which was, at one time, thought to be a temporary abnormality in some women and therefore not always treated unless it worsened. Whilst it is sometimes true that mild dysplasia may not develop beyond that stage, now that treatment is less intrusive than it used to be, most doctors take the prudent option and refer the woman for further investigations and appropriate treatment.

The next stage is what is known as "carcinoma in situ". The term itself is enough to frighten most women because it sounds so ominous. However, this is the pre-invasive stage of the disease and can be eradicated by laser treatment.

Treatment by laser is a relatively quick procedure. It is carried out in hospital, but is usually conducted in the out-patient department and so does not require an overnight stay. No anaesthetic is required, although oral painkillers are prescribed beforehand to make the procedure more comfortable. A speculum is inserted into the vagina in the same way as described for the smear test, but because the gynaecologist needs to ensure absolute stillness of his patient so that he can apply the laser accurately, the legs are held in stirrups. You therefore have to put up with this rather undignified position, but it does not last long. A special microscope called a "colposcope" is inserted so that the gynaecologist can see exactly where the problem lies and can thus aim the laser directly at that area and nowhere else. The action of the laser is to, in effect, burn the diseased cells, so the laser is "fired" in a series of short bursts. It has the effect of causing the muscles of the uterus to contract and so the sensation is similar to the heavy dragging of a period pain. I will not tell you that it is painless because it most certainly is not! The pain is not that of burning or soreness at the site of treatment, but due to the uterine contraction – an intense cramping which can be nauseating as well as extremely uncomfortable. Any amount of severe pain tends to make one feel faint, which is the body's natural inbuilt safety mechanism, blocking out pain through unconsciousness, and this procedure too, probably due more to the **type** of pain than the extent of it, is no exception.

However, once it is over, you can relax. It is followed up by a cervical smear test a few weeks later, and then again after about six months to make sure the laser treatment was successful. Occasionally, a repeat of the treatment may be required, but on the whole, once is enough. It is recommended that smear tests are performed annually afterwards, but as time goes on, if each test is negative, your doctor will probably decide that every two or three years is sufficient.

Who is at risk?

It is a disease of sexually active women, being virtually unknown in virgins, and is therefore related to sexual intercourse. It was once thought to be a disease affecting women over 40 but in fact it is common in much younger women and although it can strike at any time, the initial trigger that causes cell mutation is considered to occur at times when the cervix is particularly sensitive to change such as during adolescence or first pregnancy.

Statistically, there is an increased risk in women who have intercourse early in life, who have had several partners or who are sexually promiscuous. It is thought that it might be related to a particular chemical substance found on the head of some men's sperm. The herpes virus has also come under scrutiny, as has the contraceptive pill. At one time it was thought that there was a link between cancer of the cervix and wives of long distance lorry drivers, the conclusion being that sitting in a hot cab, on a plastic seat, especially during summer, causes sweating which in turn causes a sticky substance called smegma to build up under the foreskin of the man's penis. This smegma is thought to be a causal factor and is borne out to some extent by the fact that the disease is extremely uncommon amongst Jewish women whose partners have been circumcised.

However, whatever the "high risk" groups are deemed to be, there are always exceptions, and so one cannot afford to be complacent. There are too many grey areas and unanswered questions to feel too self-assured or convinced that because you do not fall into a high risk category, you are not at risk at all. Every woman who has embarked upon sexual activity at some time in her life, should be screened. It is the only way to truly put your mind at rest.

Fear is a great stumbling block to many things and it is a particularly active emotion when one's health is in question. Just as one might fear going to the dentist or have a fear of hospitals, some people are afraid before visiting a doctor, and so it is not uncommon by any means to feel anxious about having a cervical smear test. There may be some unknown apprehensions, for example, some people who are terrified of even visiting someone else in hospital, cannot explain why they are afraid. If this is the sort of fear that is apparent, then **ASPEN** is the remedy to help allay such vague anxiety. However, if one takes a closer look, the cause of the fear usually lies in an uneasiness about the possible outcome. Fear of cancer, or perhaps fear of the procedure itself. If the woman does not know what to expect, then the entire procedure becomes shrouded in mystery, and her imagination begins to work overtime in her attempt to speculate what might happen, and of how painful she imagines it will be. In a situation like this, when the fears are known, the remedy needed is **MIMULUS**, or **ROCK ROSE** if there is actual terror. For those wild imaginings and panic-stricken irrational thoughts, **CHERRY PLUM** is called for. **RESCUE REMEDY** however is ideal. It contains both Cherry Plum and Rock Rose, as well as **Star of Bethlehem** to relieve shock and trauma, **Clematis** for feelings of faintness and **Impatiens** for restless agitation. Four drops of **Rescue Remedy** in a glass of water before you leave the house, or whilst you are waiting, will help you feel much calmer, and if you take some with you, you can take some more drops afterwards if necessary.

The other emotion, besides fear, that can cause anxiousness is embarrassment and nervousness about being "interfered" with. **CRAB APPLE** will help if you cannot bear the thought of being examined, **LARCH** if you feel self-conscious about someone else inspecting you so intimately, **WATER VIOLET** if you are a person who keeps herself to herself and finds the process of clinical examinations too much of an invasion of privacy. If you are shy, **MIMULUS** is the remedy you need, or if you are the sort of person who seeks reassurance from others – "it **will** be alright won't it? Do you think I should go?" – **CERATO** is indicated. If however, you are troubled by uncertainty, unable to make up your own mind about whether to attend or not, but do not ask for guidance from anyone, then the remedy required would be **SCLERANTHUS**. If you are a person who tends to take life as it comes, and you feel apathetic about having the test performed – what will be will be – then **WILD ROSE** will help, or **HORNBEAM** if you procrastinate, and tell yourself "I'll do it tomorrow"!

The Bach Remedies can really help in this situation, but even more so if you are faced with subsequent investigations and treatment for a positive result. That can be an extremely anxious time and so in addition to Remedies as mentioned above, **WHITE CHESTNUT** would be helpful to settle the mind and relieve unwanted troublesome thoughts. **AGRI-MONY** is also a useful remedy for anxieties and worries if you find them hard to express and so keep them locked away inside; pretending to others that you are coping with the situation bravely and calmly and are taking it all in your stride.

If the diagnosis comes as a shock, which it inevitably will, then **STAR OF BETHLEHEM** should be taken to relieve its effects straight away. This will then take care of the worry, fear and distress that may otherwise follow. If you feel depressed then **GENTIAN** will give you encouragement, or if it is a deep gloom which portays only a picture of morbid disaster, then **GORSE** will help to restore your hope and faith in life.

To round up on a cheerful note, however, always remember that cervical cancer is preventable if caught in its early stages. There **IS** a cure, and the screening test available is a quick and easy method of making sure that you **ARE** cured if it is discovered. However, the majority of women are unaffected and so it should be considered as a means of gaining positive reassurance and peace of mind, and that in itself makes it unquestionably worthwhile.

BREAST CANCER SCREENING

With the advance in medical technology, sophisticated equipment can detect breast cancer very early, well before any physical signs become apparent. However, this diagnostic screening test, called a "mammogram" is not something offered routinely to all women. Breast cancer is more common in older women, and so mammography is generally only offered as a matter of course to women over 45. However, it can occur, albeit less often, in younger women and in particular those who have a family history of the disease, those who have never been pregnant or whose first pregnancy was after the age of 35, those who have been unable to breast feed, and those whose menstrual life has been lengthy, either due to early menarche i.e. periods started before the age of 11, or late menopause, i.e. periods continuing beyond the age of 50.

It is therefore in the interests of women of all ages, and in particular those falling into any of the above categories to examine their breasts themselves so that any abnormality can be detected and treated early. Self examination is quite simple, but first it is advisable to get to know your breasts. This way, you will not be unduly alarmed or confused by normal breast changes. During the menstrual cycle, hormones cause a number of things to happen in the body. They affect the ovaries, the uterus, and because the purpose of the cycle is for reproduction, the whole system prepares itself for pregnancy. This is why the breasts become swollen, tender or sore prior to a period – the tissues expand as they prepare for lactation. As the tissues expand, the breasts become harder and lumpier, but this is normal. To detect abnormal changes, therefore, it is best to examine your breasts when they are in a dormant phase – just after a period has finished is the ideal time because that is when the breasts are soft. If you are post-menopausal, simply examine your breasts at about the same time each month, choosing a day that you can remember easily.

The test itself is quite straighforward. You do not need any equipment, just a pair of hands and a little time on your own. First of all stand in front of the mirror and observe what your breasts actually look like. You will probably notice that one appears a slightly different shape to the other. This is quite normal. Now, raise your arms and take account of what shape they are when you have your arms extended above your head. The skin should remain smooth, so any puckering or change in appearance should be reported. Once you have examined your breasts visually, lie down on the bed so that you can examine them manually. Raise one arm above your head and then use the flats of the upper fingers of the other hand to gently feel the whole breast. Start at the outer edge and work your way round in a circle, gradually moving towards the nipple in the centre. Finally, examine your armpit, because breast tissue extends into this area too. Use gentle but firm circular movements with your hands to enable you to feel the tissues which lie under the surface of the skin. Once you have examined one breast, repeat the exercise for the opposite side.

So what exactly are you looking for? As mentioned above, the breast undergoes certain changes during the menstrual cycle, and so pre-menstrual lumpiness may be quite normal, although it is always worth asking your doctor or nurse at the clinic to reassure you. The human body is basically uniform, but each one of us has personal differences in features that make us unique. So, just as one woman may have course dark hair and another fine fair hair, so one woman may have large pendulous breasts, while another's may be small and rounded. Neither is abnormal, just different, and although it is a sad fact of life that we do not always like what we have been endowed with, it is nature, and as nature is a beautiful thing, so every woman, indeed every human being, is beautiful in their own way, whatever shape or size they might be. Similarly, just as the contour of the breast differs from one woman to the next, so the make up of the tissue within it also differs. It is therefore difficult to state cate- gorically what is normal and what is not, and because we are all individuals, we can only compare our own breasts with themselves, using our findings on the first examination as a yardstick. However, suffice it to say, that as a general rule, the breast during the first week or two of the menstrual cycle should be soft and not lumpy. A "lump" feels rather like a small hard pea or bean under the surface. You will recognize it as not having been there before and you will know it is not connected to your normal menstrual breast changes if it does not disappear with the onset of menstruation. Any lump that you find and any abnormality or change in your breast that is noticed during your own personal monthly examinations should be reported at once to your doctor or clinic nurse. The fear of finding a lump is usually what deters people from self-examination, but to ignore it is just like burying one's head in the sand. It is not going to go away, and it is important that it is investigated as soon as possible so that if it **IS** anything serious, something can be done about it without delay, and just as with cervical cancer, the sooner breast cancer is detected and treated, the better chance there is of a cure. So, if you need courage and feel afraid of what you might find, then the remedy **MIMULUS** will help you overcome your anxiety.

However, finding a lump in your breast does not necessarily mean you have cancer, so try not to be unduly alarmed. Eight times out of ten the lump will be benign – a cystic swelling or nodule which can be removed or aspirated with no difficulty. This is an important point because the natural reaction when a breast lump is found is to panic and spend the next few hours or days terrified that you might have cancer. Yet, only one lump in five is cancerous, so the chances are that you will eventually receive the reassurance that no malignant cells have been found. However, in order to determine this, you may have to undergo what is called a "lumpectomy" – the surgical removal of the tissue in question. This involves a small incision which will hardly leave a scar. The tissue will then be analysed for the presence of cancer cells.

If the results confirm that the cells are indeed cancerous, then further appropriate action will be taken to ensure that all the affected tissue is removed. If the cancer is benign, then the lumpectomy alone may well be sufficient, but this will be followed up with mammographic screening at regular intervals as a precaution in case the disease should return.

What does a mammogram involve?

It is rather like having an X-ray taken. It involves a visit to a specialised centre or to a department at your local hospital. You will be asked to undress to the waist, and then your breasts will be examined one at a time. This is not a very dignified procedure and the woman may feel very vulnerable and exposed. The machinery looks rather imposing but it simply involves placing your breast on the X-ray plate and then another section of the machine applies pressure from above. Because breast tissues is sensitive at the best of times, this part of the procedure may be rather painful, and one woman I know said her breast looked like a hamburger, sandwiched inside the jaws of the machine which she described as being rather like a trouser press! Thankfully, however, it does not take long and the results are available there and then.

Once again, it is the unknown quantity and fear related to the procedure as well as what might be revealed that presents the biggest emotional problem. **MIMULUS** will help relieve the fear; **ASPEN** the fear of the unknown; **WHITE CHESTNUT** for the worrying aspect. Here again **RESCUE REMEDY** is an ideal remedy to have by you and to take before you are due to be examined as it is, like any procedure, the thought of it and build-up before hand that is most frightening.

If results reveal that there is a malignant tumour and it is not contained within a capsule as in the case of the benign lump explained above, then unfortunately the treatment is not so conservative. It may involve surgery, radiotherapy or a combination of both. Being told that a mastectomy needs to be performed – the removal of the whole breast – is, I am sure, the news that every woman ultimately dreads. The extent of the growth determines to what extent surgery is required, and the surgeon will preserve as much of your breast as he possibly can. With plastic surgery techniques it may be possible to re-create cosmetically an acceptable breast contour. However, whatever might or might not be able to be done, it is small comfort for a woman faced with the prospect of losing a breast. It is, after all, a form of amputation, like losing a limb, and is therefore not easy to come to terms with. Careful counselling is extremely important, and if there is a partner, it is important for the couple both to be counselled, because tremendous adjustment and understanding is required so that the surgically imposed trauma does not in itself traumatise the couple's relationship. If this adjustment can begin before the operation, all the better, because it will take time, and the longer one has to come to terms with it, the easier it will be. The Remedies, although they cannot turn the clocks back or avoid what may be necessary, can certainly help you to cope and thus hasten your recovery from the trauma of the experience and this, in itself, will play a major part in your long term health and emotional stability.

Initially, shock is the biggest hurdle. **STAR OF BETHLEHEM** therefore is needed to help soften the impact of the jolt to the system the news received will undoubtedly have caused. By reducing the effects of shock, the subsequent emotional chaos is also reduced, but for the worry that inevitably follows, **WHITE CHESTNUT** is helpful as it calms the mind which otherwise tends to go round in cirlces. Fear is also apparent and a natural reaction. Nervousness will be eased by **MIMULUS**. Anxiety over the unanswered questions is eased by **ASPEN**. For a greater fear – terror, panic – **ROCK ROSE** will help to restore rationality to the mind, along with **CHERRY PLUM** if those thoughts get out of control. Before the operation and afterwards, a tremendous amount of adjustment is needed, and so **WALNUT** is a very important remedy to include as it will help the whole system to settle. The thought of being disfigured, maimed or violated is bound to occur, even before the operation has taken place, and perhaps more so afterwards when the actual reality is there staring back at you from the mirror. Many women are unable to even look. For this awful feeling of self-disgust and disfigurement **CRAB APPLE** is helpful as it re-establishes self worth and will therefore help you feel human again. This remedy is also helpful if you should feel that all eyes are on your chest; that everyone must notice that you are "deformed". It is something you are naturally going to feel self-conscious about and it is not uncommon to become paranoid about what other people are thinking of you.

For those overcome with depression, there are several remedies to consider, depending on the type of depression encountered. **GENTIAN** is for the set-back, depression for a reason; **SWEET CHESTNUT** is for an awful feeling of despair as though life is no longer worthwhile – a desperately sad feeling of having nothing to live for. Tiredness is usual after any medical treatment, surgery in particular. **OLIVE** therefore, the remedy for fatigue, is important during convalescence, together with **HORNBEAM** which helps to give strength to those who cannot find the energy to face the day ahead. Every woman's reaction will be different, depending on the type of person she is. The **AGRIMONY** woman will hide her feelings, or make light of them, make a joke about her disfigurement and conceal the tears that well up inside – tears she so desperately wants to shed. Others will react in a totally different way – perhaps needing to talk, get it out of their system, and so find themselves taking advantage of anyone who is willing to listen. This type of person needs **HEATHER** to help take her mind off her troubles. Another woman may lose confidence in herself and find it very difficult to face the world outside. This woman needs **LARCH**. Some women are naturally brave, courageous and have a resilience and solid determination to let nothing beat them. They keep on going, even when they are tired and ill, until they become physically incapacitated. For this type of person **OAK** is the remedy, and it helps to restore the natural strength to fight on. There are, however, others who are not so brave, who would become terribly despondent and give up all hope of recovery. **GORSE** is the remedy for them.

Coming to terms with mastectomy is like a bereavement, and a similar emotional process takes place. The trauma, worry and fear, particularly if suppressed, gradually turn into feelings of anger. A woman might experience a great sense of injustice and get angry because it seems so unfair. **VERVAIN** would help the frustration this causes. Or the anger may be one of hatred towards life or God, in which case **HOLLY** would be needed. It may cause a lingering and festering resentment when the mood turns inwards upon oneself and brings with it an overwhelming sense of bitterness that you are the only one who has been singled out to suffer in this way – why me? what have I done to deserve such misfortune? This feeling can soon spiral downwards and inwards, causing a build up of resentment, extending to other women who are still intact, or to one's husband or partner for "not understanding". If this is the way you feel, then **WILLOW** is the remedy to help you overcome these negative thoughts which, are terribly self-destructive and eat away at you causing a crater filled with self-pity. Willow helps that crater to fill with more positive and optimistic thoughts about yourself and others. If you feel jealous or suspicious – perhaps towards your partner or husband who, you feel, **must** despise your appearance and therefore **must** be lusting after other women, then **HOLLY** once again is the remedy to deal with these thoughts whether there is a basis for them or not.

Some women find that releasing their anger in a physical way is helpful – and indeed to off-load the adrenalin by actively getting it out of your system can be very therapeutic. Children, when they are frustrated or cross, instinctively lie on the floor with their fists tightly clenched, beating the floor with their arms and legs. By doing this, they get it all out of their system and dispose of their anger. As a similar, more adult measure (although there is no harm in beating the floor if you feel like it!), a friend tells me that a pillow makes an excellent battering ram. It causes no pain to anyone, and thus saves the aftermath of guilt which would follow if you had expressed your anger by saying something unpleasant or behaving badly towards someone you love. What is more, a pillow is totally passive and doesn't fight back!

To improve your overall health in other ways, a good diet containing plenty of fresh fruit and vegetables, preferably organic, will help your system equip itself with the vital energy necessary to repair itself and withstand the trauma. There are certain foods that are best avoided if you have had cancer, and certain eating patterns that can not only help you to recover, but help your system return to optimum health so that it is ready and waiting with all resources on stand-by should any relapse or re-invasion occur; so that you are not caught unprepared again! The Bristol Cancer Help Centre offers wonderful advice, and you may like to consider a short stay with them. You will learn a new way of life, be able to take advantage of professional counselling, gentle healing and other therapies that will, together, help you to find your own health and happiness.

== CHAPTER EIGHT ==

The Advancing Years

THE MENOPAUSE

As described in Chapter Two, a woman's reproductive life begins at puberty, at around the age of 12, with the menarche – the commencement of menstruation. It continues its cyclical pattern until about the age of 50 when she ceases to menstruate – the menopause. The term "menopause", therefore, actually describes the cessation of menstruation, but this is only one of the physical and emotional changes that take place at this time. The collection of symptoms which may occur over a period of a few years, is known as the "climacteric" and this term more accurately describes it as the change in life.

"Change" is the key-word, and this period in a woman's life demands great adjustment. The remedy that helps us to adapt to periods of upheaval and change, and therefore helpful during any major milestone, is **WALNUT**. I would therefore recommend that this remedy be included in whatever mixture of remedies you may happen to need.

It is not clearly understood exactly why the body should decide after a certain length of time, at a certain age, that it will no longer be reproductively active. Perhaps it is just nature's way of controlling human population and ensuring that the newborn and their mothers are fit and healthy. That is to say, young, which is not necessarily the same thing – there are many women over the age of 45 who are a lot fitter and a lot healthier than women half their age, but that seems to be the way nature has planned it! There is a common misconception that the menopause begins when the ovaries "run out of eggs", but this is not usually the case. The ovaries simply stop responding to stimulation from the pituitary hormones, ovulation does not occur, and gradually the follicles become less viable and begin to disappear. Consequently, there is no corpus luteum and so progesterone is absent. Oestrogen is still produced in small quantities but this too, due to the inactivity of the ovaries, is reduced considerably. The pituitary gland, however, in response to the low oestrogen levels, continues to produce FSH (Follicle Stimulating Hormone) and LH (Luteinising Hormone), and do so in vast quantities in a vain attempt to encourage the ovary to continue to ovulate. It is the reduced levels of oestrogen which are responsible for the majority of physical and, to some extent, emotional disturbances during this period of change.

Several physiological changes take place, and it is because these are associated with ageing that the menopause, in some people's minds, is considered to be the end of useful life – a turning point after which the woman goes into rapid decline; old age just around the next corner. Thankfully, this is not so. Certainly the menopause is a milestone one reaches later in life, but it certainly does not mark the finishing post. There are many more active years in anybody of that age, and especially in a woman. After all, doesn't life only begin at 40? Although a "feel better" cliche, there is a lot of truth in it nevertheless. Post-menopausal years are essentially a time when work, motherhood and home-building have been accomplished and are no longer taking up all your time. It should therefore be a "sit back and enjoy it" period. A time to rest. Often easier said than done, however, and I am sure there are many women who will agree, and attest to the fact that one's time is soon filled with other things and sometimes, one wonders whether one will really be able to sit back and enjoy it at all, or indeed, whether a woman's work is ever truly done! Nevertheless, whatever your time is or is not filled with, reaching the end of your reproductive life is a beginning of a *new* way of life, not the end of it.

It is comforting to know that two thirds of women pass through the menopause with no major problem at all, suffering with only slight symptoms, if any. But to be prepared, let us consider some of the actual physical changes, first of all, that can take place. The classic menopausal symptom is the hot flush. This may happen only occasionally, or may occur several times a day. It can be most uncomfortable, but thankfully it comes in waves and is relatively short lasting, usually only for a few minutes. It is caused by the dilatation of blood vessels in the face and neck, and because it affects the face, the one part of our body that everybody sees, it can cause acute embarrassment. It is also often followed by profuse sweating which exacerbates the problem and heightens the embarrassment. However, the flushing is not as noticeable as it feels, and so a quick glance in a mirror can be very reassuring. Hot flushes tend to be induced by excitement, anxiety or nervousness, and are quite often triggered as a result of a minor incident, especially if you are of a nervous disposition anyway. For women who suffer with nervousness and are fearful of day to day events, **MIMULUS** is the remedy to help allay that nervousness which will then go some way to easing the tension of the moment until the flush passes. It is also a good remedy for those who are naturally shy and blush easily. For those who are excitable, perhaps unable to keep still and are easily agitated, **IMPATIENS** is the remedy to restore calm and peace. **LARCH** will help the woman who feels self-conscious, feels all eyes are on her and lacks confidence in herself. **CRAB APPLE** is the remedy if you should become negatively obsessed with what you look like. Hot flushes may also occur at night, which is particularly distressing as it interferes with sleep, and because the bed-clothes are warm anyway, it is difficult to get cool, resulting in much sweating. If sleep is disrupted too much then tiredness will no doubt follow, anxiousness and worry over the prospect of it happening time after time, irritability due to insufficient sleep, and depression because it is all so wearing. **OLIVE** is the remedy to help with the tiredness, **IMPATIENS** for the irritability, **GENTIAN** for the depression.

Hot flushes however, are not the only symptom or cause of emotional upset. There is a psychological upheaval as well as a physical one, and so the emotions need time to adjust as well as the body. Emotional symptoms are numerous and vary from one woman to another. The individual personality determines the response and so the remedy or remedies that describe our character should always be included to aid a return to equilibrium. The "type remedy" is what our emotional stability rests on and so it is an important factor to consider when we are selecting other remedies to help our moods. Our whole reproductive life revolves around hormonal changes – surges of one hormone and then another, the decline of one and the increase of another. These hormonal changes – especially oestrogen and progesterone – are responsible for the emotional disharmony we encounter during puberty, adolescence and, for many women, each month during the menstrual cycle, causing the classic premenstrual symptoms of anxiety, depression and irritablity.

Because the menopause is another period of change, and because it is another major milestone, the hormonal upset is even greater and so its related symptoms are, naturally, more acute. Quite often the woman's emotions take charge and she finds herself weeping or shouting or shaking without having any control over what is happening (**CHERRY PLUM**). Some women who are normally passive and take life in their stride (eg **WILD ROSE**), become dissatisfied and intolerant of what suddenly becomes a dull and meaningless existence (eg **BEECH**). Other women who are normally active and full of life (eg **VERVAIN** or **IMPATIENS**), suddenly feel overwhelmed with lethargy and fatigue (**HORNBEAM**). Generally, women become more sensitive during the menopause and can easily take things to heart – things that they might otherwise brush off with a shrug. This may cause a certain moodiness which spirals inwards into self-pity until the woman finds herself weeping at the slightest thing. **WILLOW** is the appropriate remedy for these bouts of negativity and introspection. A woman may feel inadequate, perhaps due to the realisation that she is ageing, and naturally wonders whether her husband will still find her attractive. Women who have not settled with a partner or who are not married, might be filled with despair that the opportunity has passed them by. This again would be helped with **WILLOW** if the thoughts dwell on negative aspects of life. Married or single, for those who feel a deep sorrow at having missed out on life, or are filled with heartache when they look forward and see nothing but emptiness, **SWEET CHESTNUT** is a wonderful remedy to bring comfort to the heart. Some women may even sense a feeling of grief as though part of them has died – this sense of loss will be eased with **STAR OF BETHLEHEM**. Some women begin to doubt their ability and lack security, feel vulnerable and unable to cope with things that they used to be able to deal with easily. **LARCH** is the remedy to restore confidence, and **ELM** for the burden of responsibility – the desperate "I cannot cope with it any longer" feeling, which I'm sure is familiar to most of us from time to time! For depression there are a number of remedies. We have considered **WILLOW** for the introspective depression, and **SWEET CHESTNUT** for the heart-wrenching despair of life's future, but **MUSTARD** is another helpful remedy, and is for a feeling of depression that descends for no apparent reason, out of the blue, and is similar to the type of depression experienced pre-menstrually or post-natally. For hopelessness; a feeling of pessimism – "there is nothing that can be done for me so I may as well give up altogether" – **GORSE** is the remedy to restore hope and faith in life. If, on the other hand, the mood is one of apathy and resignation, then **WILD ROSE** is the remedy to bring sparkle back into life.

Emotional upsets and the way we feel in ourselves will, inevitably, have an impact on those around us. This can therefore cause strain in a relationship or family and then only serves to make the whole tiresome period worse. A woman who feels she is unattractive and no longer lovable may become irritable and argumentative with her husband or partner if she feels he has "gone off" her, and as a result she begins to resent him. He in turn tries to avoid such confrontations and keeps a low profile which his wife then interprets as confirmation of her suspicions which causes even more bad feeling. This situation easily gathers momentum and can cause all sorts of marital disharmony which is very sad as it is so often avoidable. **HOLLY** for the suspicion, **BEECH** for the argumentativeness, **IMPATIENS** for the irritability, **WILLOW** for the resentment and **CHERRY PLUM** for the irrationality of thoughts, all of which take charge of the mind and cause loss of control over clear straightforward thinking, are remedies that can be helpful and comforting at this time.

It is a period of adjustment for the whole family, not only the woman herself, and because her emotions can be so volatile, the rest of the family need to be extremely patient. It is not an easy time for anyone, and so much lenience, tolerance and understanding is crucial for a peaceful existence. There's frequently the tendency to blame others for their lack of understanding (**WILLOW/BEECH**). Whether or not there is any true basis for feeling this way, these remedies would apply if the mood is apparent. Of course, if other family members, husband, partner etc., are finding it difficult to be sympathetic and understanding, then the remedies are there to help them too, depending on their needs. One further remedy which may prove helpful is **SCLE-RANTHUS**. Although the remedy is primarily for indecision, it can be very useful for any form of imbalance, and because the moods can be so volatile, swinging from one to another, Scleranthus helps to bring stability to those fluctuating emotions.

Other problems which might upset your relationship with your partner are those associated with your sexuality. The reduced levels of oestrogen causes the lubricating secretions of the vagina to gradually diminish and for some women this results in dryness and soreness, particularly noticeable during intercourse which sadly, may become painful and unpleasurable. It can, however, be easily overcome by the use of a lubricating gel, and **Rescue Remedy Cream** is also very soothing. However, this problem is more common in older women, and so although it may **begin** at the time of the menopause it is not usually noticeable until much later on. Whilst on the subject of sex, there is an unfortunate and quite unrealistic mode of opinion that there is something unnatural about an older woman having sexual desire. As a consequence the older woman with her wholly natural sexual needs, may feel she is perverse or abnormal and so becomes embarrassed or ashamed. This is the sad result of ignorance on the part of those who generate and uphold such a narrow-minded view, and not the fault of the woman concerned. She is merely the victim of society's prudery. It may be, perhaps, the result of the common misguided view that sexual desire is related to fertility. This is not so. Sexuality and the fulfilment of sexual needs goes on right into old age, and contrary to public opinion, it is the man who finds age interfering with both his desire and his performance as he gets older, and this is often the main reason for a decline of sexual activity in later life.

The natural physical changes taking place during the menopause – greying hair, wrinkles, an increase in weight and distribution of fat from where it was once used to enhance features to places where it is least appreciated – all act as evidence that the ageing process is taking place, and it is then with dismay that the menopausal woman sees her young body being replaced with something that looks, to her, unattractive and undesirable. This in itself may cause her to question her sexuality. However, during the menopause, a woman's sex drive may actually increase, and many women find that sex is more fulfilling than it was in their youth – not necessarily through sexual intercourse itself, but through gentle body contact, hugging, cuddling and a general growing closeness and feeling of warm togetherness. Like a good wine, a woman's sexuality tends to mature with age!

HYSTERECTOMY

It seems appropriate to discuss this subject here as, although it is not related to the menopause or climacteric directly, and is not necessarily confined to women in later life, it does present difficulties in its own right, and some of these are similar to those experienced during the menopause.

Hysterectomy is the removal of the uterus or womb. It does not necessarily mean the removal of anything else. The vagina remains intact and the ovaries are preserved whenever possible. Occasionally they may also require removal and if so, then the menopausal symptoms will result due to the enforced reduction in ovarian hormones – oestrogen and progesterone. These symptoms can, however, be relieved by hormone replacement therapy which may be particularly helpful for the younger woman undergoing this operation.

There are a number of reasons for performing a hysterectomy. It is not always due to cancer. It may be due to fibroids or because of a menstrual disturbance that cannot be resolved any other way. A woman who is advised she needs a hysterectomy however, needs careful counselling so that she understands what is going to happen and why, and can be reassured about issues that may be worrying her.

The loss of this very female organ may make a woman feel that she is no longer complete – no longer a real woman – and this feeling can be most alarming and disturbing. Gentle reassurance and guidance, however, can help greatly to allay fears and re-build confidence and understanding.

Here again, sex is another worry which is often expressed. Many women believe that they will no longer be able to have intercourse, but this is not so. The vagina is not affected and so there is no physical reason why a normal sex life should not be resumed. Sexual arousal and ultimate fulfilment is not affected by the removal of the uterus. It is, however, the emotional aspects that are responsible for most difficulties experienced in the continuation of a happy sexual relationship. **CRAB APPLE** will help the woman who feels she cannot bear the thought of being "incomplete" and begins to hate herself. This remedy will also help the woman who cannot bear the thought of sex or her husband/partner touching her. **MIMULUS** will help the woman who is afraid. Frequently, these two states of mind go hand in hand, in which case both remedies would be required.

Although hysterectomy is an operation most commonly performed on women approaching the climacteric or who are post-menopausal, occasionally, due to medical reasons, it may be deemed necessary for a much younger woman. If she has not already had a family or feels her family is not yet complete, it presents an obvious difficulty and may be disastrous for her. If children are dearly wanted, it can be devastating to be told that one will never be able to experience motherhood, and although there are ways and means of having a family through adoption and surrogacy, it is not the same as carrying your own child. The grief and despair are soothed with **STAR OF BETHLEHEM** and **SWEET CHESTNUT**. **PINE** would help the woman who feels guilty or blames herself, perhaps feeling she is depriving her husband of fatherhood or not being able to fulfil her feminine role completely.

However, hysterectomy is not an operation performed for no reason at all. If at all possible, an alternative treatment will be offered. This being the case, the condition that makes the operation necessary would be something that has been causing a lot of discomfort, pain, or heavy periods, and so in the long term it should come as a relief – freedom from annoying and uncomfortable symptoms.

EMOTIONS IN LATER LIFE

We start ageing from the moment we are born, but it is not something one really thinks about until much later in life. When a woman reaches perhaps her thirties or forties she might begin to consider the ageing process as something looming ever nearer, especially when she begins to notice the odd grey hair or "crow's foot" under her eyes! These signs which tell us that we are mellowing become more and more apparent as time goes on. It is something that happens gradually until the menopause when the whole process seems to speed up. The reason for this is hormonal – oestrogen is responsible for so many things that are associated with youth, that when our oestrogen levels begin to wane, youth too begins to elude us. This is why hormone replacement therapy (HRT) is often advocated, at least for women whose lives would be otherwise intolerable. However, whilst it certainly helps a number of women, it does not suit everyone, and when it is prescribed, its administration is carefully monitored as side effects are not uncommon in women taking synthetic oestrogen.

Oestrogen is responsible for the elasticity of the skin and so as the level of this hormone drops, the skin loses its elasticity, hence the wrinkles, flabbiness, sagginess and breasts that start to droop. It also causes the skin to become thinner, which means that areas which have little flesh such as shins and knuckles tend to be more prone to injury if they are knocked. **RESCUE REMEDY CREAM** is therefore handy to put in your first aid box, if it is not there already! In addition to this, thinning of the skin affects the lining of the vagina so that it may become sore and dry. Again, **Rescue Remedy Cream** may prove helpful. Oestrogen also affects the bones, and when the level is very low, reduced calcium levels result in a degeneration of the bone tissue, causing bones to become brittle. This condition is known as Osteoporosis and occurs in about 20% of women over the age of 65. It tends to be diagnosed or becomes apparent if a woman suffers a fracture. In the elderly, falls can result in a fractured neck of femur, the bone of the hip which because of its situation, is particularly vulnerable.

Sometimes osteoporosis may be diagnosed if a woman complains of back pain which may be the result of a vertebra wearing or "collapsing". This is what causes elderly people to appear to shrink with age. If you should happen to suffer with pain in your back it would be advisable to seek the advice of a qualified chiropractor; a specialist in the manip-ulation of spinal displacement. All our nerves emanate from the spinal cord and so pain or discomfort anywhere in the body could be due to some misalignment of the spine and can often be solved by the gentle manipulation of chiropractic. Women who are post-menopausal would be well advised to ensure their intake of calcium is adequate by either taking calcium supplements or a calcium-rich dietary intake of foods such as milk.

So, how does all this affect our emotions? Once again, women vary. Some do not mind getting older. Certain physical conditions might be a nuisance, but otherwise it is a natural process and so they feel comfortable with it. For other women, it spells disaster. The sight of an old woman peering back at them from the mirror where once a young face looked out, can be most depressing. Once again those feelings of being "past it", unattractive and undesirable creep in, and it may be a time when a lot of reassurance from friends and family is needed. In addition to this, as old age creeps nearer, there are emotions attached to the reality of life drawing to a close. Once again this can take a lot of getting used to, and if it all seems rather unsettling **WALNUT** is the remedy to help ease the transitional adjustment. It may also come as rather a shock; a sudden realisation that the last chapter of one's life may have arrived, and for this **STAR OF BETHLEHEM** will help to relieve the emotional trauma of such a revelation and sooth the mind in this respect.

A lot of fear may also be apparent, filling the thoughts with apprehension about what is to come. This may be fear of illness for which **MIMULUS** would be the remedy to help relieve such anxieties, or there might be fear of incapacity which again would be helped with **MIMULUS**, but in addition to this, there may be a feeling of guilt – feeling a burden to other members of the family, or worry about how one is going to manage. A sense of guilt would be helped with **PINE** and **WHITE CHESTNUT** for the worry and mental turmoil that so often accompanies it. If there is anxiety over others, afraid of how **they** will manage or what effect coping with your ill-health might have on their lives, **RED CHESTNUT** is the remedy to help you to see the situation realistically and in proportion. Fears and concerns of this nature are uppermost in the minds of many ageing women, and because of the nature of their emotional upset, they often keep it all to themselves and do not ask for help or talk it over with their family, simply because they do not want to be a nuisance and do not want to worry them. Once again **RED CHESTNUT** and **PINE** would be appropriate, along with **AGRIMONY** for the inner worry and turmoil that is concealed behind the bright "oh yes I'm fine; don't worry about me dear" remarks. For women who are brave and solid, and although their physical body might not allow them to do all the things they would like to do, do not give in to the ageing process; those who keep on going and remain young at heart, **OAK** would be indicated. This is a very positive remedy as people of this nature have an in-built resilience and strength. However, Oak people, being the way they are, feel even more frustrated and unhappy if they are incapacitated, so although they do not tend to worry about the prospect of becoming ill – they have an "I'll concern myself with that when the time comes" approach – if and when it does, their remedy **OAK** will help them to find their inner strength should it temporarily desert them, to look ahead patiently to the day when they will be back on form, and until then accept that they must rest.

Advancing years may also cause lethargy, lack of energy or resignation to life's consequences. **HORNBEAM** is the remedy required for the lethargy and will help provide more strength to look forward to the day ahead with more interest and enthusiasm. **OLIVE** is indicated for mental and/or physical tiredness when there is little energy left to carry out even pleasurable activities. **WILD ROSE** would be indicated if resignation and apathy have taken over, acceptance with one's "lot", content to sit back and watch life pass by. Often elderly people worry about lack of sleep and ask for help because they are not sleeping as well as they used to. Sleep problems and insomnia may be due to worry or fear and so remedies appropriate to these needs would be required, but it is not always appreciated that as one gets older, sleep patterns change. We need more sleep during periods of growth – childhood, adolescence, pregnancy and during lactation. In later life, our need for sleep is reduced and so only five or six hours may be sufficient whereas eight or nine were a "must" in more youthful days. If this is not understood, it can cause a great deal of anxiety, and also, if a person is in the habit of taking an afternoon "nap", then the need for sleep at night will be reduced even further. There are practical measures which one can take to help relieve the "problem", but often it is the understanding of one's need for less sleep that will help to settle those who are anxious. If it troubles you, **WAL-NUT** would help you to adjust to this new way of life, or new way of sleeping. But once you can appreciate that it is normal not to sleep for such a long period, then waking up at night need not be such a frustrating and worrying event. People I have spoken to frequently say that they feel wide awake in the early hours of the morning, or they do not feel tired when they retire to bed at what is deemed to be "bed-time". The thing to do is to find something to occupy your mind – read a book or get up and make a hot drink or do the crossword in the paper. My mother does the ironing, or prepares a meal for the following evening!

As our lives advance, there is more accumulated behind us

than lies ahead of us, so it is only natureal that we look back on all the happy memories and re-live past events. These memories may be happy ones or they may be sad, or what is usual, a mixture of the two. There may be regrets or un-fulfilled dreams, wishing one could turn the clocks back and do things differently. For feelings like this, **HONEY-SUCKLE** helps to bring the attention back to the present so that the past can be reflected upon without becoming all-consuming. If there is resentment about a missed oppor-tunity or towards other people or events that have made you unhappy, **WILLOW** is the remedy to help you put such feelings behind you, so that you can forgive and forget. **WALNUT** too may be a useful remedy to consider as this will help the adjustment to life's changes, and although ageing is not something that happens suddenly, there is nevertheless a settling down period at each milestone, when we have to get used to new ways and put the past behind us. This is where Walnut helps as it makes that transition from one way of life to another that little bit easier.

Jane Evans, author of "An Introducton to the Benefits of the Bach Flower Remedies", has written numerous articles for the Bach Centre's newsletters. The following was pub-lished in March 1976, but like the Bach Remedies themselves, it is a timeless piece of writing and I hope that the subject, being so relevant to this chapter, will appeal and be of help.

"Surrounded by problems, as we are in this world today, by worries, anxieties and pressures of every kind, some people find it very difficult, as they get older, to relinquish.

The rather desperate desire to put off as long as possible, to refuse to hand over responsibility to youn-ger people, to change habitual working routine, can be, indirectly, an appeal for help. They become emotionally distressed, fears and depression creep in. They may even become possessive and irritable. They are vulnerable, knowing that soon changes will have to be made, but they can only see the losses entailed, not the gains.

Should we be in the position to help anyone with such difficulties of adjustment perhaps a few general suggestions might be of use, for a little sympathetic attention at this time could lead them to come to appreciate the value of the Remedies through the help they themselves have received at a time when hopelessness for the future might have set in. With **GORSE** to change the hopelessness and lift the depression, the attitude should be more encouraging.

As people grow older, usually a slowing down process takes place which can be resented. If this is at all evident, **IMPATIENS** for the irritability of frustration, and **WILLOW** for the resentment. No longer making frequent contact with former colleagues, with the previous work-pattern broken, can bring about a feeling of loss of status, for which **LARCH** would help to regain the necessary confidence to embark on some new enterprise.

The physical aspect of advancing years may well require a change of emphasis, of energy, switching to the development of other latent abilities. Following this may be a time of indecision, wondering which new interest to pursue. If this is the difficulty **SCLE-RANTHUS** should help to dispel the doubt. Some clear indication could then be determined. Or if there is confusion, through the over-generous advice of friends, then **CERATO** would resolve the situation.

New contacts made through increased leisure may, and probably will, suggest new outlooks and further ways in which the Remedies can help ourselves and others in need by meeting requirements as occasions arise. With the emphasis more on "advancement" than "age", the positive aspect will soon clarify. Soon the incoming interests will exceed the time available, then the negative aspects become reversed.

Let us try to encourage people we know with retirement problems by helping them to see that it really is a progressive rather than a retrograde step, a time to develop more enlightened thinking, a time of awareness of profound simplicities – which is indeed the message of the healing flowers we use."

DEATH AND DYING

Perhaps one of the hardest things to come to terms with is the prospect of dying, coming face to face with one's own mortality as it looms ever closer the older we get. Some people cannot bear the thought of it at all and will do anything, take anything or eat anything in an attempt to arrest the ageing process. The anxiety connected with this way of thinking however, is its own worst enemy and can in itself cause the very things that one is trying to escape from. However, remedies can help in this respect too. **MIMULUS** for fear; **ASPEN** for the fear of the unknown, trepidation over the unknown element of what lies ahead; **ROCK ROSE** if there is terror. There is, of course, nothing wrong with keeping fit and healthy, looking after oneself, taking regular exercise, keeping a check on weight, taking care of the skin etc. Naturally, this is a good thing to do as it will undoubtedly improve the quality of life, giving the body the best chance possible to withstand disease and incapacity later on, or to be on top form to recover quicker and with more efficiency than we might otherwise have done. It is only when the desire to keep well and stay healthy becomes an obsession and causes anxiety or tension that we need a little help – the Remedies will not deny us the enthusiasm or drive to help ourselves, but will help us to be more relaxed about it so that it really does have some lasting good.

Coming to the end of life, however, is as natural as being born. Our physical body will not, we know, go on forever. One day we will die, which is about the only thing in life we can reliably count on! We do not know when it is going to happen, we do not know how it is going to happen, or whether we will live until we are 99 or 29. Yet, the life we live as a human being is not our entire life span. It may be all we can relate to as a person with a name and title, living within a family in a particular place, doing a particular job. But if you accept that there is more to life than our earthly existence, then True Life is eternal.

This idea may not, however, be acceptable to everyone – some may not be able to see beyond the boundaries of the physical existence that we experience as a human being.

However, I have often looked up at the stars on a clear night, as I am sure many others have done, and tried to imagine infinity. We are told, and science has confirmed it, that the solar system, galaxies and the universe go on and on and never end. To fully appreciate that concept is really not possible – the human brain is simply not capable of comprehending infinity. But if we really think about what is around us, if we think about the stars and the whole marvellous cycle of life, how it all fits so neatly together, then it is difficult to conclude that there can be nothing more to it than this life. There **must** be more, otherwise what would be the purpose in it all?

> "The short passage on this earth, which we know as life, is but a moment in the course of our evolution, as one day at school is to a life, and although we can for the present only see and comprehend that one day, our intuition tells us that birth was infinitely far from our beginning and death infinitely far from our ending. Our Souls, which are really we, are immortal, and the bodies of which we are conscious are temporary, merely as horses we ride to go on a journey, or instruments we use to do a piece of work."

Edward Bach, Heal Thyself

There are so many things in life that we do not understand, and probably never will, but that is because we are human, and thus it is part of our learning during this particular chapter in our evolution. If we came into this world equipped with all the answers, then there would be nothing for us to learn. We would gain nothing from our existence here. To quote Dr. Bach again, "We are not permitted to see the magnitude of our own Divinity, or to realise the mightiness of our Destiny and the glorious future which lies before us; for, if we were, life would be no trial and would involve no effort, no test of merit. Our virtue lies in being oblivious for the most part to those great things, and yet having faith and courage to live well and master the difficulties of this earth. We can, however, by communion with our Higher Self, keep that harmony which enables us to overcome all worldly opposition and make our journey along the straight path to fulfil our destiny, undeterred by the influence which would lead us astray."

So, there are certain aspects of life that we do not know, things we have to have faith in and simply believe. We believe in radio waves yet we cannot see them, feel them or capture them, yet our radio and TV set picks up the signal. That signal, the music or the picture, is our proof that those waves are really there, and we continue to believe they exist even when the radio or TV set is switched off. Unfortunately we do not all have "spiritual radios" that we can turn on to provide us with proof of the existence of our soul or the life that awaits us, but there are some who do have such a gift and are sensitive to the energy of life, and some may share that insight with others. Whether it be a psychic gift or the gift of healing, we all have it to some extent, although some people are more sensitive to it than others. Our intuition is our Higher Self speaking to us and guiding us, if we will but listen.

"Everyone of us is a healer, because every one of us at heart has a love for something."

Edward Bach, Free Thyself

Nora Weeks was Dr. Bach's closest colleague, and during the years she spent with him during his search for the remedies got to know his work thoroughly and became an extremely good friend and support. She continued to prepare and send out the Bach Remedies for over forty years after Dr. Bach died, together with their other companion Victor Bullen. Nora Weeks was 82 when she died in 1978. She had a few bronchial problems but otherwise she was generally fit and healthy, although perhaps a little physically frail during her latter years. Nevertheless, she worked until the end and always kept herself fully occupied – gardening, reading, writing, as well as the day to day correspondence and general running of the Centre. She lived at Mount Vernon, and the work was her life. She was a remarkable woman and thankfully remained mentally astute all her life. Her memory and the care she took in her work was impeccable.

Nora never married, although she always had companionship – Victor Bullen and, of course, Dr. Bach whom she loved and respected deeply. She kept her personal feelings very much to herself and in the true spirit of a thoroughbred Water Violet, always referred to him as "Dr. Bach" or "the Doctor". Never did she refer to him as "Edward". Dr. Bach's work filled every moment of her life. She had very little time to be bored and because she was in close contact with many very good friends, never had the chance to feel lonely. Perhaps in her quieter moments when she could be alone with her thoughts, uncertainty or apprehension might have reared in her mind – she was, after all, left in charge of the future protection of Dr. Bach's work which was an enormous responsibility for her, and although she had Victor's moral support, Nora ultimately bore it all. She was, however, an emotionally strong woman and she simply followed her intuition and what she knew Dr. Bach wanted, remaining absolutely true to her convictions. The Remedies were of course, always there to help her, and I'm sure she had Dr. Bach's gentle presence to guide her, but her faith in truth meant that she was never in any doubt

As Nora got older, she never became frightened of death. To her it was a natural progression – another step forward. One very good friend, Henry Moorhouse, who had known Nora for 35 years, wrote a tribute to her in the Bach Centre Newsletter shortly after she died. He said "To Nora, 'passing on' was merely removal to another sphere of healing and to a fuller knowledge of Dr. Bach and all the joys associated with the Remedies."

Indeed, she believed that her life as "Nora Weeks" was only part of a much greater life and although she enjoyed every minute of it, learning and experiencing and fulfilling the tasks set for her, she looked forward to her own passing with excitement, and just as a sailor who had been at sea for several months would be filled with a calming joy at the sight of his homeland appearing on the horizon, to Nora leaving this earthly plane was like returning home after 82 years away!

WIDOWHOOD

Statistically, women live longer than men and so in older age it is more likely that a woman will be on her own for the latter years of her life, than will a man. Coming to terms with the prospect of losing one's husband or partner generates all sorts of emotions – fear, anxiety, panic, sadness, despair. Fear of loneliness, of managing, coping on one's own; worrying about dealing with everyday affairs; sadness at the thought of one's partner no longer being around; and despair at the inevitability of it all. However, if possible, we tend not to look ahead too far or dwell on these unhappy thoughts. We try to put them to the back of our mind, preferring to deal with it when the time comes and enjoying a life together now. Indeed, dwelling on morbid thoughts achieves very little. It does not make it any easier to bear when the time does eventually arrive, and it means that the present is forsaken which is a great pity. Nevertheless, if these thoughts do cross your mind, as would only be natural from time to time, the Remedies can help you to put them into perspective and bring the present back into positive focus once more.

MIMULUS – for fear

ASPEN – for apprehension and a feeling of uneasiness

ROCK ROSE – for panic and great fear

WHITE CHESTNUT – for worrying thoughts and restlessness

SWEET CHESTNUT – for the despairing anguish.

One day, however, it might be that you are alone, your husband or partner having predeceased you. We have discussed the emotions surrounding the prospect of our own death, and really the same applies to the death of our loved ones. Nevertheless, no matter how philosophically we might look at it, losing someone dear and as close as a husband or partner is that much harder to bear. Grief can seem to follow a bizarre pattern in some instances, but these moods and emotions are natural. The series of feelings pass through stages, and there are a number of these, lasting different lengths of time for different people. Grieving – being able to cry, offload the emotion, scream, lash out or whatever, is a release, and as such, a normal and very natural part of healing. We are all individuals and so we all react in our own individual way; how we deal with our own grief and pain is a personal thing. Sometimes it is helpful just to be alone with our thoughts, to be able to think about one's loss, think about the person no longer by our side, and all the memories that will be cherished forever. Some people find it very difficult to express their feelings, even to themselves, and thus try to block the thoughts from their mind, and as a consequence feel that they have never really grieved; never cried. This may be interpreted as bravery, but for most, it is a suppression of feelings and because the grieving process is a natural one, re-establishing inner peace and equilibrium, to miss out on it is, in effect, missing out on an important aspect of that healing process. However, everyone copes with it in different ways, and so each one of us needs time in which to express and come to terms with our own pain. What is right and helpful to one is not necessarily right for another. Shock, and the series of emotions that result from it can get "blocked" and the tears that are so desperately awaited to relieve the shock, fall inside instead of out, drowning the pain and causing even more emptiness. It is sometimes the feeling of numbness that stops the tears from flowing, but when they do, although the heartache comes too, it does at least mean that at last the grieving process and thus healing is beginning.

The Bach Remedies help to ease the emotions by helping you to find your own way through it. They do not suppress the feelings because this would be to stifle them, but rather, they allow you to tackle each stage as it comes more positively and with more certainty, and just as though you were on an ocean voyage in a small boat in a storm, guide you safely to your destination and help keep you afloat so that your boat does not sink and place you in danger.

STAR OF BETHLEHEM is the most important remedy initially, but it is helpful at a later stage too, whenever the effects of shock are still apparent. It is the comforting remedy in times of sorrow and thus helps to ease the grief and emptiness.

HONEYSUCKLE – this remedy will help those whose minds dwell on the past. However, thinking about happy times, reminiscing and remembering places, people, and occasions that have been shared together are not thoughts that will want to be replaced. They are your memories and will be there in your mind to comfort you and keep you company. Why then, should Honeysuckle be needed? The remedy is there to help if, instead of gently reflecting, your whole mind is locked away in the past, preventing you from progressing on your own journey in life. Often, memories are linked to sorrow as well as happiness, and so Honeysuckle in this sense will assist Star of Bethlehem in its work of repair and healing.

SWEET CHESTNUT – this remedy is for the anguish felt at the thought of the future when nothing but emptiness lies ahead; when life no longer seems worthwhile. Sweet Chestnut is a wonderful remedy to uplift the heart and soul and offer, once more, a guiding torch to show you the way through what seems to be a dark and dismal tunnel of life ahead.

WILLOW – a number of people have said that they feel angry and resentful towards their loved one for leaving them alone. This remedy helps you to realise that it was not something done with intent to hurt, but just a cruel fact of life. Willow also helps those who begin to resent life, wonder why **they** have had to suffer, and so, as they think about and reflect upon their own grief and unhappiness, find their thoughts beginning to become more and more introspective, becoming an unstoppable spiral of sorrow, resentment and self-pity. Again, this is a natural emotion and nothing to feel ashamed of. Many people who feel this way feel guilty as well, but if the mood is presenting itself as a stumbling block then Willow is the remedy needed to help lift that obstacle out of the way so that the passage forward becomes clearer and brighter.

PINE – this remedy is for those who feel guilty; perhaps blame themselves for not having foreseen an illness or tragedy, or for not having done more. This may be especially apparent for those who have lost someone through an accident or sudden illness. Guilt may also cause a great deal of self-reproach if, for example, your husband or partner's death came suddenly and you never had the chance to say goodbye. Or it may be that he met with a fatal accident or collapsed whilst out, and before he left the house you may have quarrelled, leaving each other under a cloud of bad feeling. For the guilt that so often follows, Pine is a very helpful and comforting remedy.

VERVAIN – this remedy will help ease the sense of injustice at life for having been so unfair. It is for the tension and frustration associated with having had something snatched away from you in an unreasonable or unjust manner. This feeling may be associated with resentment so would, in that case, be combined with Willow, or it may be associated with hatred in which case Holly would be a helpful complement to ease the anger.

HOLLY – this is for emotions such as hatred, desire for revenge, suspicion or envy. It is not uncommon to feel angry, even hate the person you have lost for having left you; for being so selfish as to die and leave you alone, and it is certainly not uncommon to feel hatred towards life itself for being so wicked. Envy, jealousy or even hatred towards other women who still have a living partner is another common and normal feeling. For all these emotions, which can sometimes be quite violent in nature, Holly will help you to cope and reverse the negativity.

ELM – for those who feel suddenly overwhelmed with the responsibility of looking after the household, money, the car, the repairs. Although many women have shared the home-maintenance and stereotypic "male jobs" around the house, there are equally many women who have not, and so do not have the practical experience required to turn their hand to leaking taps or burst pipes. Something which may in itself be quite trivial can therefore seem like a disaster. Elm is the remedy to help you stay abreast of it all and restore confidence and faith in yourself.

GENTIAN – when things go wrong and discouragement and despondency descend, Gentian is the remedy to help lift the spirits and help you bounce back and try again.

HORNBEAM – this remedy will help if you feel you do not have the strength to face the day ahead. If you feel tired before you begin, weary at the thought of getting through another twelve hours, Hornbeam is the remedy to give you the strength to face it all, and more enthusiasm for what is in store.

WHITE CHESTNUT – for worrying thoughts or mental arguments. These troublesome thoughts may cause insomnia and restlessness at night, and if so, White Chestnut will help to release the mind from the events of the day, or the worry of tomorrow, and thus restore calm so that sleep naturally follows.

MIMULUS – for fear of worldly, everyday things. It is the remedy to give courage to those who are nervous or afraid.

WATER VIOLET – for those who bear their grief silently; those who do not, or feel they cannot, talk to others; those who become isolated, when friends and neighbours may feel awkward or uncertain about how to make their approach, and for the loneliness that may result. This remedy will help you to share your pain, find a shoulder to cry on and find again that quiet peace.

A MAN'S PERSPECTIVE

So far we have concentrated on the woman's feelings connected with either the thought of losing her husband or partner, or the reality of bereavement and widowhood itself. However, we have not mentioned the feelings of the partner.

He too might be afraid (**Mimulus**), perhaps guilty for leaving his wife alone (**Pine**), or may worry and fear for her well-being (**Red Chestnut**).

Victor Bullen, close friend and companion to both Nora Weeks and Dr. Bach had a beautiful philosophical outlook on life and he was able to offer a gentle guidance to many, many people. I hope that by repeating his thoughts here, entitled "Young Old Age", that gentle guidance will help many more for years to come, and be a comfort to women who face losing or who have lost a husband, parent, brother, sister, companion or close friend:

"One is glad to have lived long enough to enjoy old age. One learns to adapt oneself. Although more slow in thought and action, one may still enjoy this thrilling adventure of life here on earth to the full. Indeed, the enjoyment is more keen so long as one does not spoil the "here and now" by foolish and futile regrets in respect of the past and depressing fears for the future.

One is so happy still to be able to enjoy things. Even the morning shave is something to be lingered over with pleasure instead of a bore. The chores, the grates, the washing up, the weeding, all become part of the glorious adventure of life, instead of the trivial round to be endured. One can so easily become the prey to dark thoughts and ill-health if the mind is not filled with interest and love of life. Just as fear and expectance of ill-health lower vitality and attract diseases, so fear of old age attracts its crippling limitations, one can become paralysed with terror. Joy **OR** fear are more infectious than measles. So that whilst health remains we can still serve and communicate joy simply by ourselves remaining serene and happy.

What of the future? There comes to me a recurring dream when I stand and watch the inexorable tide flowing towards me. A moment of apprehension when the flood carries me away and there is nothing but the vast grey ocean, and then the thrill of being lifted and carried towards a glorious sun coming up over the horizon. A glimpse of infinite beauty and peace beyond telling. A breath-taking dawn chorus, the warm welcome of friends.

There is no death."

Further Suggested Reading

BACH FLOWER REMEDIES

The Twelve Healers & Other Remedies – Edward Bach
Heal Thyself – Edward Bach
The Bach Flower Remedies Step by Step – Judy Howard
Questions & Answers – John Ramsell
Handbook of the Bach Flower Remedies – P. M. Chancellor
Dictionary of the Bach Flower Remedies – Tom Hyne-Jones
The Medical Discoveries of Edward Bach – Nora Weeks
The Original Writings of Edward Bach – Judy Howard &
    John Ramsell
Introduction to the Benefits of the Bach Flower Remedies –
    Jane Evans
The Bach Remedies Repertory – F. J. Wheeler
The Bach Flower Remedies Illustrations & Preparations –
    Nora Weeks & Victor Bullen

> All the above published by the C. W. Daniel Co. Ltd.

The Story of Mount Vernon – Judy Howard, Bach Centre.

Bach Flower Therapy – Mechthild Scheffer
    Thorsons Publishers Ltd.

Flower Remedies to the Rescue – Gregory Vlamis
    Thorsons Publishers Ltd., 1986

OTHER SUBJECTS

Aromatherapy for Women – Maggie Tisserand
    Thorsons Publishers Ltd. 1985

Getting Pregnant – Robert Winston
    Anaya Publishers Ltd. 1989

Natural Fertility Awareness – John & Farida Davidson
    The C. W. Daniel Co. Ltd. 1986

Everywoman – Derek Llewellyn-Jones
    Faber & Faber Ltd. 1971

The Vegetarian Mother & Baby Book – Rose Elliott
    Fontana Paperbacks 1984

The Bristol Programme – Penny Brohn
    Century Hutchinson Ltd. 1987

Natural Pregnancy – Janet Balaskas
    Sidgwick & Jackson Ltd. 1990

The Book of Yoga – The Sivananda Yoga Centre
    Ebury Press. 1983

Pregnancy – Gordon Bourne FRCS FRCOG
    Pan Books Ltd. 1984

First Baby After Thirty – A Marshall Cavendish Publication,
    Consultant Editor Roger V. Clements FRCS (Ed).,
    FRCOG
    Windward, 1986

You Can Heal Your Life – Louise L. Hay
    Eden Grove Editions. 1984

Useful Addresses

The Dr. Edward Bach Centre
Mount Vernon,
Sotwell, Wallingford,
Oxon. OX10 0PZ (advice and information about Bach
Flower Remedies)

The Dr. Edward Bach Foundation,
Dr. Bach Centre,
Mount Vernon,
Sotwell, Wallingford,
Oxon. OX10 0PZ
(education, training and registration of Counsellors in the
Bach Flower Remedies)

Bach Flower Remedies
6 Suffolk Way,
Abingdon, Oxon. OX14 5JX
(general information and orders)

Nelsons Homeopathic Pharmacy,
73 Duke Street,
London. W1M 6BY
(Nelson and Bach mail order)

British Homeopathic Association,
27a Devonshire Street,
London. W1N 1RJ

The Tisserand Institute,
65 Church Road,
Hove, East Sussex. BN3 2BD
(Aromatherapy training and register of practitioners)

Aromatherapy Products Ltd.,
Knoll Business Centre
Old Shoreham Road,
Hove, Sussex. BN3 7GS
(books and essential oils)

The London Lighthouse (for sufferers of AIDS)
111–117 Lancaster Road
London. W11

The Institute of Pure Chiropractic,
14 Park End Street,
Oxford. OX1 1HH
(Register of McTimoney Chiropractors)

The Bristol Cancer Help Centre,
Grove House,
Cornwallis Grove,
Clifton, Bristol. BS8 4PG

Frank Roberts (Herbal Dispensaries) Ltd.,
91 Newfoundland Road,
Bristol. BS2 9LT

The National Marriage Guidance Council (Relate)
Herbert Gray College,
Little Church Street,
Rugby. CV21 3AP

Breast Care and Mastectomy Association of Great Britain,
15–19 Britten Street,
London. W3 3TZ

Womens Mid-Life Centre,
Birmingham Settlement,
318 Summer Lane,
Newtown, Birmingham. B19 3RL

National Association for the Childless,
The Birmingham Settlement,
318 Summer Lane,
Birmingham B19 3RL

Foresight (Association for the Promotion of Pre-Conceptual
Care)
The Old Vicarage,
Church Lane,
Whitley, Godalming, Surrey. GU8 5PM

SANDS (Stillbirth & Neonatal Death Society)
Argyle House,
29–31 Euston Road,
London. NW1 2SD

British Pregnancy Advisory Service,
Austy Manor,
Wootton Wawen,
Solihull, West Midlands. B95 6BX

National Council for One Parent Families
355 Kentish Town Road,
London. NW5 2LX

British Association for Counselling,
37a Sheep Street,
Rugby, Warwickshire. CV21 3BX

National Institute of Medical Herbalists,
P.O. Box 3,
Winchester, Hants. SO23 8AA

Iyengar Yoga Institute,
223a Randolph Avenue,
London. W9 1NL

British Wheel of Yoga,
1 Hamilton Place,
Boston Road,
Sleaford, Lincs. NG34 7ES

The Sanctuary (health club – a truly unique experience!)
11 Floral Street,
Covent Garden,
London. WC2E 9DH

Index

Using the index

Each emotion or state listed refers you to a Remedy (e.g. aloofness to Water Violet) and under the name of the Remedy you will find entries for various situations in which that emotion may occur. There are many ways of describing feelings such as aloofness: reserved, self-contained, un-approachable, keeping yourself to yourself, private, isolated, lonely, inhibited, detached, unmoved have all been used in this book. To keep the index as clear and concise as possible I have used only the definitions in the list of Remedies on pages 4–7 with a few additions where there is a substantial piece of information.

When using the index please do look up the page reference as the full description of the state that is given there will help you decide exactly which Remedy suits you.